The IMG's Guide to Mastering the USMLE & Residency

NOTICE

The IMG's Guide to Mastering the USMLE & Residency

Keshav Chander, M.D.
Fellow, Department of Cardiology
Alton Ochsner Medical Foundation
New Orleans, Louisiana

McGraw-Hill
Health Professions Division

New York St. Louis San Francisco Auckland Bogotá Caracas Lisbon London Madrid
Mexico City Milan Montreal New Delhi San Juan Singapore Sydney Tokyo Toronto

McGraw-Hill

A Division of The ***McGraw-Hill*** *Companies*

The IMG's Guide to Mastering the USMLE & Residency

1234567890 PBTPBT 99

ISBN 0-07-134724-0

This book was set in 12 point Goudy by V&M Graphics, Inc.
The editors were John Dolan, Susan Noujaim, and Barbara Holton.
The production supervisor was Rohnda Barnes.
The cover designer was Janice Barsevich Bielawa.
The index was prepared by Jerry Ralya.
Phoenix Book Technologies was printer and binder.
This book is printed on acid-free paper.

Library of Congress Cataloging-in-Publication Data

Chander, Keshav.
The IMG's Guide to Mastering the USMLE & Residency—1st ed.
p. ; cm.
Includes bibliographical references and index.
ISBN 0-07-134724-0
1. Physicians, Foreign—United States—Handbooks, manuals, etc. 2. Residents (Medicine)—United States—Handbooks, manuals, etc. 3. Medicine—Examinations—Study guides. I. Title: The IMG's guide to mastering the USMLE & residency. II. Title.
[DNLM: 1. Foreign Medical Graduates—United States. 2. Internship and Residency—United States. W 20 C454u 2000]
R697.F6 C45 2000
610.69—dc21 99-054041

To my father
the late Shri Mehar Chand;
my ever-inspiring son Girish; and to
two great women, my mom
Mrs. Krishna Wanti and my wife Renu.

Acknowledgement

Thanks to medical students and residents from American medical schools and the IMGs whose experiences and fears were responsible for this book.

I gratefully acknowledge the contribution of the following (in random order) toward the making of this book:

- IMGs, my friend Dr. Srinivas Koya and my wife Dr. Renu Mahajan for their constant advice and feedback.
- IMGs from different parts of the world who filled out my survey. Their phenomenal enthusiasm to get all this information out to other IMGs was a constant inspiration to me.
- My teachers, Professor of Medicine, Amritsar Medical College, Dr. R.K. Kumra and Chief of Cardiothoracic Surgery at Escorts Heart Institute New Delhi, Dr. N. Trehan.
- K.S. Sandhu and his family for their support through my initial months in the United States.
- Mr. Darren Barré for helping me with the photographs in the book.
- Dr. Preston Cannady, Jr., Internal Medicine program director at Chicago Medical School for his support through initial stages of this book.
- My fellowship program director Dr. Tyrone Collins, Chairman Dr. Christopher White, Vice Chairman Dr. Richard Milani and Cath lab Director Dr. Stephen Ramee at Alton Ochsner Medical Foundation for providing the right atmosphere for me to write a book in the very first year of my fellowship.
- Dr. Donald Erwin, Director of Graduate Medical Education at Alton Ochsner Medical Foundation for his encouragement throughout the process of writing this book.
- Mr. Martin Wonsiewicz, Publisher, McGraw-Hill, Inc., Health Professions Division for his help through the initial stage of the book.

- The Executive Editor Mr. John Dolan for his invaluable advice and help in giving a concrete form to my idea.
- The Development Editor Ms Susan Noujaim for all her help and advice.
- Editing Supervisor Barbara Holton and all the others at McGraw-Hill who were involved with creation of this book or getting it to the readers.
- Dr. Herman Price, Dr. Mark Cassidy, Dr. V. Chilakamarri, Mr. Gregory Bodin and Professor Tumulesh Solanki for helping me with different sections of this book.

I am grateful to my parents, my brother Ashok and sisters Usha, Geeta and Sneh for supporting me through all my endeavors.

Contents

Who Should Buy this Book?

- IMG physicians who are at different stages of receiving training in the United States:
  - Those in their own countries who have ever thought of going to the United States for training.
  - Those in their own countries who are having jitters about going to the United States embassy for a visa application.
  - Those in their own countries or in the United States who are at different stages of taking the different qualifying tests.
  - IMGs anywhere in the world who are interested in doing a residency in the United States.
  - IMGs who are already at different stages of residency in the United States (from internship through the stage of planning for a fellowship after finishing a residency).
  - Those engaged in the hunt for a good fellowship.
- Members of the public worldwide who may be interested in knowing how they can help a friend or family member at one of the stages enumerated above.
- Educators worldwide who are interested in knowing more about residency training in the United States.
- Health care professionals in the United States who are interested in understanding residency training in the United States from an IMG's perspective.

Preface

Welcome to the exclusive club of doctors who have ever dreamed of making it to the United States for training. As a general rule, doctors in any country are people of at least above-average intelligence. It takes a certain amount of discipline and strength of character to secure a slot in medical school and survive the grind after getting there. After all the years they have to put in, it is only fair that doctors be allowed to dream of and work toward the pinnacle of their desired goal. This book has been written to guide you in the process of getting into residency training in America and doing well once you are there.

People who were ready to go the extra mile to achieve their goals built the United States as a country. This is a country that has always been ready to embrace the very best of the world. This means two things. First, this country never closes its doors tight to outsiders in case one of them is a potential Nobel-prize or Olympic gold-medal winner. Second, the onus of convincing the authorities that you have solid potential is on you.

Unlike many potential immigrants who are ready to do so-called "odd" jobs in America, you, as a doctor looking for residency training in the U.S., have a well-demarcated market. However, it takes a lot of planning to make the journey to your goal a smooth one. Good planning can mean the difference between getting into an elite university or a small hospital in a God-forsaken place or, worse still, not getting a residency position at all. If you do make it into a residency program, your future depends entirely on how well you do in the residency, because in the American health care system, no one moves forward without good recommendations from the people he or she does the residency with. Having the proper information is the key to successful entry into and completion of a residency in the United States.

To date, international medical graduates (IMGs) planning to come to the United States have been basing their actions on information received in bits and pieces from different sources. Based on their sources of information, I have divided them into the following groups:

1. IMGs who have a sibling or a very close relative who is a doctor in the United States.
2. IMGs who have acquaintances in the United States, but whose acquaintances have no first-hand information about the field of medicine in the United States.
3. IMGs who have a close friend or a casual acquaintance in the medical profession in the United States.
4. IMGs who get information from IMG chat rooms on the Internet and try to extrapolate someone else's experience to their own situation.
5. IMGs whose only source of information about America has been Hollywood movies or perhaps a single visit to the United States Information Agency (USIA) in their country. Once you start looking around you, you will be surprised at how large a percentage of people belong to this latter group.

The problem with depending on any of these sources of information is that (1) they may not have the information that you require or (2) their information may be tinted by an occasional incident specific to a particular individual's life.

Among the observations that led to the inception of this book are the following:

- Many IMGs come to the United States with little useful information and lots of raw enthusiasm. This can lead, and has led, to tragic failures after arrival in the United States.
- Many concerned parents of IMGs are very anxious at the thought of their child going off to the United States. Most give in to the dreams of their starry-eyed child. Such parents can gift this book to their child and feel satisfied that they have done their bit to help smooth their path.
- Some IMGs end up with low scores on the U.S. Medical Licensing Examination (USMLE), making it difficult for them to get into a residency program after coming to the United States. This can throw them into a state of perpetual hopelessness.
- Some IMGs fail the USMLE, Clinical Skills Assessment (CSA), or English exams repeatedly.
- There is little literature discussing the problems faced by IMGs trying to come to or survive after coming to the United States for training. Many review books are available to help students studying for the exams, but IMGs need to know more than that.

- IMGs have to work hard to learn many of the things that sound commonsensical to someone who has grown up or done a clinical clerkship in the United States.

This book is written to help you plan your entry into a residency program in the United States in the new millennium. The goal is to ensure that you do not have to settle for anything less than what you deserve. The residency slots available to IMGs have been shrinking. This book will give you a head start over your competition. Before you can be eligible to do a residency in the United States, you have to pass the USMLE Steps 1 and 2, Test of English as a Foreign Language (TOEFL), and CSA exams. This book will help you understand what you need to know to be able to do well on these exams.

The computerization of these exams, as well as the residency application process is likely to make things more difficult for some IMGs who may not have much experience with computers. I have discussed ways to use computers for the intended task at different points in this book.

This book provides information on how to get into a residency program and how to do well once there. It is important that you know a considerable bit about the experience of residency in the United States at an early stage for these reasons:

1. IMGs trying to take the USMLE exams come across the following caution time and again: "IMGs must get a high score to be able to better their chances of getting a residency in the United States." In the absence of any other suggestion, the only thing left for them to do to achieve a better score is to study "harder." Most IMGs study their best before taking this expensive exam, but the statistics show that the pass rate for first-time exam takers is about 90% for U.S. students versus a dismal 60% for IMGs. I think one important but little talked about factor influencing the pass rate is the need to be able to read and understand long vignettes well in order to do well on the exams. The vignettes are written to reflect the types of scenarios that you would encounter in U.S. hospitals. To better understand them, you should either have done a clerkship in the United States or have some knowledge of the working style of doctors in U.S. hospitals.
2. As a part of the CSA, you will be evaluated according to the American system. To pass this test, it is important to know the

way medicine is practiced in the United States. There are some significant differences in history-taking as well as management of patients in the United States as compared to other countries. These are discussed in detail in this book.

3. You need other basic information well in advance to be able to do your best in a residency program in the United States. Once you get into the residency program, the new work and social culture will place tremendous demands on you. You may be overwhelmed by seemingly insignificant things, finding the secrets of success in the residency only after it is too late. This lack of advance knowledge can thus seriously hurt your career prospects or family life. Some examples of the things you need to know:

   a. How to prepare for work as an intern in a busy hospital in the United States. Most of the time you will have to hit the track running with not much orientation time. This can wreak havoc on you, physically and mentally.
   b. How to obtain medical care for you and your family
   c. How to get a fellowship
   d. How to plan your return to your own country after training
   e. How to carry out efficient job search in the United States

This book is probably the first attempt to empower IMGs with all of this information. I do not know if any book can tell you anything to assure 100% success, but I am sure that nothing in this world assures 100% failure. Ignore your nonmodifiable weaknesses and start working on your strong points. This book should help you do that.

You have already proven your intelligence by getting into medical school. You are flexing the muscle of your ambitions by thinking about entering a training program in the United States. Now join me in the journey through the intimate secrets of residency training in America. In this day and age, the person with more and better information is the winner. And this book is my effort to make you one. Happy journey!

Keshav Chander, MD

CHAPTER 1

Evaluating Yourself

During my stay in the United States, I have seen hundreds of international medical graduates (IMGs) coming here from different countries. Most of these people come to the United States believing that they will have access to all the modern technology for treating their patients. Some of them are motivated by stories of doctors living in million-dollar mansions, but nearly all of them have neglected to step back and evaluate themselves before coming. It is extremely important to be aware of your characteristics so that you can exploit your strong points and work on your weaknesses.

By the time a person reaches the United States, he or she falls into one of the following groups:

1. Fresh graduates who are driven by their peers in medical school. There are medical schools in some countries where almost the whole class takes the U.S. Medical Licensing Examination Step 1 (USMLE 1) en mass in the third year of medical school. Later the same batch takes the U.S. Medical Licensing Examination Step 2 (USMLE 2) after the final year. Some in this group catch the next plane to the United States after graduation day. These people either have a close acquaintance in the American medical profession or have resourceful parents or relatives. On average, most people have spent a few postgraduation years in their own countries before coming to the United States.
2. People who have achieved a high level of training in their own country.
3. People who have gained recognition in their own country, some of whom may be internationally known. Interviews with some of these people reveal a common denominator: While

they were successful according to the standard definition in their society, they were not according to their own definition.

4. People who come to the United States for a short period of training.

GROUP 1

If you belong to group 1, your strengths are abundant energy and lots of enthusiasm. Some program directors prefer fresh grads, thinking they are easier to break in. IMGs in this group are statistically less likely to have a family and children. This means they are more likely to be ready to spend extra time in the hospital, something a lot of senior doctors love.

There is a downside to being in this group. These people enter a foreign culture with raw enthusiasm. A lot of them have not yet learned the art of covering their deficiencies. Depending on whether they hit it off with the people at their workplace, they can fly or flop. Another danger is that being young, these people can easily lose focus and forget their reason for coming here. People in this group should have a concrete plan about taking exams and finding a residency before they come to this country. This book will help IMGs in group 1 come up with a solid plan of action.

GROUP 2

Those who belong to group 2 may have a good market for their skills. Many programs prefer candidates with previous training because those candidates are ready from the word go and are capable of handling a big patient load. The going at the workplace will be much easier for them because they have a solid fund of medical knowledge and can devote a lot of time to getting used to the new culture. Depending on the type and level of training, they may be able to complete their training in less than the normally required time. For example, one may be able to finish internal medicine residency in 2 years instead of the normal 3 if one can provide evidence of 3 years of training in internal medicine in the native country. This has to be accompanied by proof of continuing satisfactory performance in the residency program in America. For further information on the criteria for this special consideration, contact the

American Board of Internal Medicine (ABIM) by calling 1-800-441-2246 or visit its Web site at *http://www.abim.org.*

There are some negatives to belonging to this group. The experience of internship can be very painful for someone with previous training and expertise who is asked to run errands and not talk back. Also, every time you get trampled by a colleague, you will think about the great things you could have done in your country with your level of training.

As a solution to the first problem, you should know what being a resident means. It is easier to handle problems you already know about and this book can help you do that. As for the second problem, make a list of things that helped you make the decision to move so far from home. This has to be done before you come to the United States and has to be done in writing. Once you have written it on a piece of paper, put it in a safe place and later, in your baggage. Once you come to the United States, you will be looking at your own country from a distance and that distance will generate a lot of love and patriotism. Here are a few examples of this phenomenon:

- That tight-lipped poker-faced professor in medical school suddenly looks like a great man with superhuman clinical sense.
- You start longing for all the members of the family who you avoided when you were back home.

GROUP 3

Those belonging to group 3 have to take stock of the situation before coming here. Using the model of a typical person in your situation, let me analyze the situation. Your major responsibilities are likely to be your spouse and children. You will almost be starting your life again. You may be one of the older residents in your cohort. This means that you do not have a lot of time to waste; that is why you need to jot down every detail of your itinerary before coming to America. You will be able to get by on the basis of your knowledge of the medical field, but the experience of residency may be difficult and painful. People in this group should do some homework before embarking on the journey. Try to cut a deal with an institute as far as the number of years of training required and the posttraining scenario. To do this, you will have to approach an institute that appreciates your previous experience. For example, if you have done significant research on human immunodeficiency virus, you should not approach a hospital interested predominantly in cardiology. As a general rule, you should approach academic institutions, not community hospitals for which a high volume of satisfied patients is the most important way of breaking even. See if you can make your potential employer see some grant money Health and Human Services (HHS) money. HHS is a government agency that gives millions of dollars in grants to institutions to do research. For information about this agency, visit the Web site at *www.hhs.gov* or call (202) 629-0257. Once you have someone interested in you, you can negotiate better to get your prospective employer to sponsor a better visa for you. When you walk into the office of a senior staffer at an institution, the responsibility for showing your potential is entirely yours. Most institutions will go to great lengths to help you once you get them interested.

Some people in this group, believing in their desirability, come with bag and baggage to the United States before securing a spot. This takes away their ability to walk away from a deal they do not like. I will discuss various types of visas in Chapter 2.

GROUP 4

People in group 4 are the elite and normally have no problems in the beginning. They have a specific period of time during which they have to be in the United States. They have everything set up before coming here and typically come without a lot of responsibilities. All this helps them stay focused and work hard during their stay. However, this group is uniformly ignorant of the rights of aliens in the United States. This makes them work harder than they have to. Being aware of the temporary nature of their visit, they are ready to tough it out anyway, but awareness of their rights can help them get more out of their visit.

The problems for these people start when they think about changing from a temporary stay to a permanent one. This means taking exams, staying in a foreign country, and wiping the slate clean to start over. This may put some people back a decade or more. In the beginning you may think that you will never do this, but look around. As a solution to this problem, secure a good job before coming. Write down all your strong points, including your own and your family's position in your country. If you still decide to try to get into an American residency, you should create a timetable for all the steps needed to practice as a doctor here. Many people blindly take this path. Later, they start thinking about all the great things they could have done if they had returned home immediately after training, but it may be too late by then.

THE NEEDS OF YOUR FAMILY

Regardless of the group you belong to, you must think about your spouse's needs if you are married. If you have a working spouse, you must do some research on his or her prospects. This can prevent frustration and heartbreak later. If you have children, you must plan ahead for their schooling and upbringing. Private schools are very expensive in the United States, and you may not be able to afford them on a resident's salary. The standard of public schools (schools that are funded by federal, state, and local government) varies between locations. The quality of schools in a particular locality is one of the major factors that determine property values in that area. This may help you understand the importance of knowing about the quality of schools when you are looking for a place to live. Typically, you will not have as much social support in your new community as you have in your own country.

OUT OF TOUCH WITH MEDICINE FOR A WHILE?

As the preceding discussion illustrates, once you start working seriously toward getting into a residency in America, you have to take a number of steps. Some IMGs may stop working while still in the home country to study for the USMLE. Others may need a few years after coming to the United States before they become eligible for residency, during which time they are out of touch with patient care. Some program directors look suspiciously at such candidates. Some state licensing boards also demand extra documentation from these IMGs.

Try to stay in touch with patient care before coming to the United States. This is even more important since the introduction of the Clinical Skill Assessment (CSA) examination. Try to tailor your style so that you can do well before trained examiners. The human cases on which you will be tested will be prototypes of typical American patients. It will take a little focused training with a specific orientation before you can do well in this test. The best way is to practice with real patients. You may have some difficulty getting involved in actual patient care (even under strict supervision) once you are in the United States because of legal and availability issues. If you are already in the United States, try to do an observership in a hospital and make sure that one of the attending physicians documents the fact that you have worked with him or her. In some states, you can also do an externship. That means you can be involved in patient care under strict supervision.

Some IMGs in the United States choose to do research while waiting to pass the exams or get a residency, thinking that this will help them get into a residency. In my opinion, this is useful only in these situations:

- You do research with the person who is directly responsible for making the decision about giving residencies.
- You are pretty sure you will get a high-quality paper published during the period you plan to work.
- You are doing research with a well-recognized authority.

With the introduction of CSA, it may make more sense to do an observership that will give you time in the patient care area. Getting an observership is difficult for three reasons:

1. You will not be helping the people you work with, as you will not be allowed to do anything connected with actual patient care.
2. You are one extra, unsophisticated body roaming around in the hospital who could become a legal liability.
3. You may be a nuisance if you start asking a lot of questions when the rest of the team wants to rush through the rounds after a busy on-call night.

As part of the solution to these problems, I suggest that you approach someone for an observership through a contact who works in that hospital or knows the people who matter. If you do not have that option, walk through the hospital door with all your charm switched on.

The person accepting you for an observership is doing you a favor. It is your job to make the team feel comfortable and safe in your presence. This can be done by being nice to the team members and being aware of the limits of your involvement in patient care. Once you are in, you may feel you are a passive member of the team. This, combined with the desire to impress the people around you, may stimulate you to get involved in patient care more than it is legally safe to do. Do not do that. You can help the team by looking up the answers to the questions that come up during the rounds and help the interns and residents look up an article that they may want to present in the daily morning report. In this way, you will be sharing the load with them, on the learning side at least.

If you cannot get an observership, another way of staying in touch is to go to different teaching sessions, such as the morning report or noon conference of a residency program. It will be easier to get permission to attend these sessions. You can even get permission for this at the chief resident level, but try to get it from the main decision maker in the residency program. This way, that person will be aware of your presence in the teaching sessions. This may come in handy when you interview at the same place for a residency. Sometimes you may be able to get a recommendation letter on the basis of this limited contact. Attendance of teaching sessions also will help you prepare for exams by teaching you the American approach to patient care.

WHY DO YOU WANT TO GO TO THE UNITED STATES?

Many doctors reach America in a twilight state. Most of them give a stereotypical answer to the question of why they came. It is very important to define your primary goals. Awareness of your primary goals will guide your actions. Look at this checklist:

I want to be in America because

- ❑ I will enjoy my life there.
- ❑ The future of my children will be better.
- ❑ I want to make a lot of money.
- ❑ I want to reach the academic heights in my chosen field.
- ❑ This is the only country where I can have a good life and also have professional satisfaction.
- ❑ I am here for training and will return to my country to practice medicine after that.

Depending on your main reason for coming, you will have to do a reality check. This means you have to do some research on whether you will be able to achieve your primary goals by coming to the

United States or would be better off staying in your own country. Most people feel blessed when they hear that they have been accepted in a training program in the United States. In the heat of the moment, they forget to analyze the situation. I have seen people who set out with the intention of learning intraocular lens implantation and found themselves instead in an institute whose strong point is posterior chamber surgery. Also, you may end up in a program where teaching has a very low priority.

If you are coming here for the money, you may be in for a surprise. While you will make a very comfortable living, undue expectations can leave many IMGs feeling frustrated later. Another important reason for going through this checklist is that each goal will demand different actions.

GOAL SETTING

TIMETABLE FOR EXAM PREPARATION

After you have decided to apply for a residency in the United States, you have to make a timetable for the different steps required. People who are already in the United States and those who have just decided to make their dream a reality should do this.

It is a common practice among medical students to sit down and do heavy-duty cramming 2 months before the exam, but by the time you take the USMLE, your responsibilities may have changed. Here is a description of the tests you will take.

USMLE 1

This examination tests your knowledge of the basic sciences. Basic sciences are typically an ignored field in medical school. If you are still in medical school and are serious about getting to the United States, take this test as soon as you have been tested on these subjects in medical school. For a person already out of medical school, I recommend at least 6 months of serious studying.

USMLE 2

This examination tests your knowledge of clinical medicine. Unless you have been studying with the USMLE 2 specifically in mind, you may not do well in this exam at the time of graduation from a non-U.S. medical school. I recommend 6 to 9 months of serious USMLE-oriented study before taking this test.

Clinical Skill Assessment (CSA) Examination

Read the rest of this book before you think about taking this test. If you are still in your own country, start to practice interacting with patients and other colleagues as described in this book. If you are already in the United States with no chance of going back to your country before taking this test, modify your thought process in accordance with the suggestions in this book. For people still in the home country, taking the CSA is a very expensive venture, and currently Philadelphia is the only place where you can take it. You will have to fly to the United States and spend a few thousand dollars to take a test you are not sure of passing. Needless to say, you want to be very well prepared.

USMLE 3

This test is not a prerequisite for getting into a residency, but you will have to take it if you want to get into residency on an H-1 visa or are already on an H-4 visa because of your spouse. You cannot work on an H-4 visa, and so you have to convert it to H-1 before you join a residency. The only way to be eligible to do that is to take the U.S. Medical Licensing Examination Step 3 (USMLE 3) before interviewing for a residency.

After you have the Educational Commission for Foreign Medical Graduates (ECFMG) certificate, you have to start applying for a residency, then go to interviews, then wait for residency match results, and then do the paperwork, for the lucky ones that get residency.

This process may take between 1 and 2 years in the best possible scenario. You have to have that much time at your disposal before you start to prepare for a residency position in the United States.

PROFESSIONAL GOALS

It may seem odd to examine this topic before thinking about an actual residency. Most of you are reading this book before getting into a residency, but it is very important to know about your goals. If you want to get where you want to be, you have to be ahead of the game.

That means you have to work on fitting into the mold according to the market forces.

It is very important to set your goals right at the start. You have to be very clear about what you want to do after residency, including the following areas:

- Subspecialty training
- Returning to your country for practice
- Private practice
- Academics

You will have many infatuations along the way, but this book will help you stay focused and prevent you from wasting time on things that do not fit well into the framework of your plans.

If you want to go into practice, you have the following options:

- Solo
- Group practice
- Working for a health maintenance organization (HMO)

A solo practice means you have your own practice. You are on call for your patients day and night. Solo practitioners are turning into an extinct species, because they have to compete with huge HMOs. If you happen to be one of the lucky ones who are not under the threat of being wiped out by that competition, you may have the pleasure of having full control over the care of patients. If that is your goal, try to learn about all the primary care topics. Try to learn as many procedures as possible. These should be procedures that a primary care physician is allowed to do in a private practice. For example, there is no point trying to learn endoscopic retrograde cholangio-pancreatography if you are not planning to specialize in gastroenterology. Try to learn as much about the diseases that are common in the population you are going to serve as possible. This is called "learning bread and butter stuff" in American slang.

If you want to go into a solo practice, you will have to have close relatives who have been in the country for years because you need a patient population that will be ready to come to you when you finish your residency. Alternatively, you should have family members or friends who are practicing in different fields and can supply a small group of patients to keep you afloat while you build your own patient base.

In a group practice, a group of doctors practice together. Another option is to work for an HMO. These organizations prefer a jack-of-many-trades. They may expect you to be able to take care of patients in different age groups, especially in the outpatient setting.

If you want to get into academics, make sure you know why. If teaching is something you enjoy, this may be right for you. Your life is likely to be less hectic if you are working in an academic institution because you will have a long line of residents and fellows working for you. In America, most doctors in academics also practice patient care. This is a safer bet, because if you are in academics purely for research, you depend on grant money and must keep the grant dollars coming. This may not be entirely under your control. Moreover, with the changing nature of the American health care system, research dollars have been shrinking.

Specialist or Generalist?

A lot of IMGs come to the United States in a search of academic excellence, and becoming a subspecialist is a part of that endeavor. Cardiology seems to be a particular favorite with IMGs from the Indian subcontinent. There has been a lot of talk about an oversupply of specialists lately. The trend toward doing a fellowship still exists among IMGs despite the fact that most American graduates go into primary care. Study the market forces at the time of your training, as they keep changing. You should do what you love to do because that is what you will end up doing throughout your life.

As a corrective measure for the oversupply of specialists, fellowship slots have been cut down and the duration of hot fellowships such as cardiology and gastrointestinal medicine has been increased to 3 years from 2. An intended effect of these measures is that fellowships are difficult to come by. Whenever something is rationed, IMGs feel the effect of cutbacks first. Fellowship hunting is one of the areas where advanced planning pays maximum dividends (see Chapter 14).

If an IMG wants to return to his or her country, he or she should try to gain expertise and maximum confidence in the field of training. Once an IMG goes back to her or his country, she or he will be expected to be an authority in that field. People in this group should create a strong network of specialists in America before going home. You can fall back on these people if you have any questions while practicing in your country. This is a symbiotic relationship. You get some names to drop among your local peers and your American counterparts have the satisfaction of being an expert before an international audience.

SUMMARY

Before going on to the next chapter, do the following:

1. Stand back and see if you fit into group 1, 2, 3, or 4. Make a checklist of your strengths and weaknesses.
2. Make special efforts to avoid being out of touch with medicine for a prolonged period.
3. Set up a timeline for completing all steps required to get into a residency in the United States.
4. Clearly visualize your professional goals.

CHAPTER 2

Getting to the United States

Among all the steps IMGs need to take, gaining entrance into the United States appears to be the rate-limiting step for most aspirants. If you are not already in the United States, you will have to come here to take the CSA and then return once more for residency interviews. The final step occurs when you return to enter a residency program. The type of visa you have for your residency can decide the future course of your stay in the United States, and so planning is of paramount importance. Table 2–1 enumerates general tips you need to know regardless of the type of visa for which you are applying.

It is very important to know about these issues because most of you will travel to get to the consulate in your country. It is very frustrating to be stuck in another city without a photograph or money order or bank draft. I have been told by some IMGs that "entrepreneurs" stand outside the U.S. consulates in some countries. They will offer to get you a photograph and even a money order or bank draft on the spot for a phenomenal sum. It will be a tragedy if that draft or money order turns out to be fake. The consulate officials try to drive such con artists away, but it is difficult to obstruct a deal between an aggressive seller and a desperate buyer.

"ACHIEVING" THE VISA—STRATEGIC MOVES

Every applicant seeking a visa is presumed a potential immigrant unless the applicant takes steps to suggest otherwise.

Fear of being refused a visa engulfs almost all IMGs who go to a consulate. You will hear "horror" stories of applicants who have been refused a visa. Various guesses (that I have no reason to believe) are as follows:

- "That blond counselor (or that lady counselor with the long nose) always refuses or issues the visa." IMGs sometimes travel hundreds of miles to another consulate to avoid a particular counselor.

- "It is better to go to the embassy at the start of the week because they exhaust the quota of nonimmigrant visas (NIVs) towards the end of the week."

Anyone who claims he or she can influence a counselor's decision is trying to con you. In reality, the only thing these people charge for is filling out a simple application form. They have no control over events beyond that. Being a doctor, you should not need to pay someone for helping you with an NIV.

REFUSAL OF THE VISA—SECTION 214(b)

It is important to understand Section 214(b) of the Immigration and Nationality Act to understand why some people are refused an NIV

Call the nearest U.S. consulate office in advance to find out about the paperwork needed to apply for the visa.

TABLE 2-1. Tips for Obtaining a Visa to Enter the United States

1. Have your passport ready well in advance. This is the first essential step toward being able to travel abroad. Acquiring a passport may take different amounts of time in different countries, in different states of the same country, and even in the same country at different times.
2. Call the U.S. consulate office in your country well in advance before going there to apply for a nonimmigrant visa. Ask them about the following things:
   a. The paperwork you will need to bring along for the type of visa you intend to apply for.
   b. Whether the embassy is open on the day you plan to go there. The local U.S. consulate may be closed on certain local and U.S. holidays.
   c. The fees involved. You will have to pay a nonrefundable service fee set in U.S. dollars. As you are likely to pay this in your local currency, it may change with the fluctuating exchange rate. You will have to know various modes of payment acceptable to the consulate: money order, check or draft, and so on. This fee is nonrefundable whether you get the visa or not. The citizens of some countries may have to pay more money once they are granted a visa. The fee may differ according to the duration and the type of the visa issued.
   d. The photographs you may have to present.
   e. Optional documentation that may help you obtain your visa. The official may or may not be willing to answer this question.
   f. Limits on the number of applicants the local consulate deals with every day. If a limit exists, you should go to the embassy a few hours in advance to get a place in the line.

again and again while others walk in and effortlessly come out of the embassy with a visa in hand. This knowledge will help you better prepare to apply for an NIV. The following text contains excerpts from the official Web page of the U.S. Department of State:

> Section 214(b) is part of the Immigration and Nationality Act (INA). It states: Every alien shall be presumed to be an immigrant until he establishes to the satisfaction of the consular officer, at the time of application for admission, that he is entitled to a nonimmigrant status. . . .
>
> To qualify for a visitor or student visa, an applicant must meet the requirements of sections 101(a)(15)(B) or (F) of the INA respectively. Failure to do so will result in a refusal of a visa under INA 214(b). The most frequent basis for such a refusal concerns the requirement that the prospective visitor or student possess a residence abroad he/she has no intention of abandoning. Applicants prove the existence of such residence by demonstrating that they have ties abroad that would compel them to leave the U.S. at the end of the temporary stay. The law places this burden of proof on the applicant. Our consular officers have a difficult job. They must decide in a very short time if someone is qualified to receive a temporary visa. Most cases are decided after a brief interview and review of whatever evidence of ties an applicant presents.

WHAT CONSTITUTES "STRONG TIES"?

Learn what constitutes "strong ties" and work toward demonstrating them.

Again, the U.S. Department of State notes:

> Strong ties differ from country to country, city to city, individual to individual. Some examples of ties can be a job, a house, a family, or a bank account. "Ties" are the various aspects of your life that bind you to your country of residence: your possessions, employment, social and family relationships.
>
> Our consular officers are aware of this diversity. During the visa interview they look at each application individually and consider professional, social, cultural and other factors. In cases of younger applicants who may not have had an opportunity to form many ties, consular officers may look at the applicant's specific intentions, family situations, and long-range plans and prospects within his or her country of residence. Each case is examined individually and is accorded every consideration under the law.

As this excerpt makes clear, you will have to prove that you have reasons to go back to your country. The onus of proving the point is on you, and you have very little time to do that; thus, good preparation and good communication skills will come in handy. The importance of appearing before the counselor well rested and well prepared cannot be overemphasized.

TYPES OF VISA

Below, I will explain the requirements for different visas. This book is not intended to be an exhaustive description of the immigration process. Information given here is meant as a rough guide and should not replace expert legal advice. Rather, I will enumerate some helpful points regarding the visas that most IMGs are likely to need (Table 2–2).

TABLE 2–2. Types of Visas
B-1 visa
J-1/J-2
H-1/H-4
Immigration

B-1 VISA

This is the visa that you will generally need to obtain when planning to come to the United States to take the CSA, and later, for residency interviews. The B-1 is the nonimmigrant visa for persons who intend to visit the United States temporarily for business. In your case, the "business" will be taking the CSA or appearing for residency interviews. The following text is based on the official Web page of the U.S. Department of State.

QUALIFYING FOR THE VISA

Applicants for visitor visas to the United States must show that they qualify under provisions of the Immigration and Nationality Act. The presumption is that every visa applicant is an intending immigrant. Therefore, applicants for visas must overcome this presumption by demonstrating that:

1. The purpose of their trip is to enter the United States for business. *In your case, you will have to present the documentation of your registration for the CSA or the interview call letters.*
2. They plan to remain for a specific limited period.
3. They have a residence outside the United States as well as other binding obligations that will ensure their return abroad at the conclusion of the visit. *The binding obligations that ensure your return to your country could be in the form of strong family ties, material possessions, or your employment with a well-respected institution in your country.*

Applying for a Visitor Visa

Applicants for visitor visas should apply at the American embassy or consulate with jurisdiction over their place of permanent residence. Although visa applicants may apply at any United States consulate office abroad, it may be more difficult to qualify for the visa outside the country of permanent residence.

Required Documentation

Each applicant for a visitor visa must pay a nonrefundable application fee (US$45 at the time of writing of this book) and submit the items listed in Table 2–3.

TABLE 2–3. Documentation Required to Obtain a Visa

1. An application Form OF-156, completed and signed. Blank forms are available without charge at all U.S. consular offices.
2. A passport valid for travel to the United States and with a validity date at least 6 months beyond the applicant's intended period of stay in the United States. If more than one person is included in the passport, each person desiring a visa must make an application.
3. Two photographs 1 and 1/2 inches square (37 × 37 mm) for each applicant, showing full face, without head covering, against a light background.

A person whose passport contains a previously issued visitor visa should inquire about special expedited procedures available at most consular offices for issuance of a new visitor visa.

- Unless previously canceled, a visa is valid until its expiration date. Therefore, if the traveler has a valid U.S. visitor visa in an expired passport, he or she may use it along with a new valid passport for travel and admission to the United States.
- If there is a fee for issuance of the visa, it is equal as nearly as possible to the fee charged to U.S. citizens by the applicant's country of nationality.
- Applicants for visitor visas should not find it necessary to employ others to assist them in preparing documents or securing access to the U.S. consular office.
- Attempting to obtain a visa by the willful misrepresentation of a material fact, or fraud, may result in the permanent refusal of a visa or denial of entry into the United States.
- If the consular officer should find it necessary to deny the issuance of a visitor visa, the applicant may apply again if there is new evidence to overcome the basis for the refusal. In the absence of new evidence, consulate officers are not obliged to reexamine such cases.

The duration of your stay in the United States is decided by INS officials at the port of entry, not by the consulate issuing the nonimmigrant visa.

U.S. Port of Entry

Applicants should be aware that a visa does not guarantee entry into the United States. The U.S. Immigration and Naturalization Service (INS) has authority to deny admission. Also, the INS, not the consular officer, determines the period for which the bearer of a visitor visa is authorized to remain in the United States. At the port of entry, an INS official must authorize the traveler's admission to the United States. At that time, the INS Form I-94, Record of Arrival-Departure, which notes the length of stay permitted, is validated. This process can be confusing if you are not prepared for it. When you enter the United States, you should be ready to explain to the INS officials at the airport how long you intend to stay and why that length of stay is required. The length of stay permitted will be the one noted on your I-94, not the duration of validity of your visa.

Visa Waiver Pilot Program

Travelers coming to the United States for tourism or business for 90 days or less from qualified countries may be eligible to visit the United States without a visa. Currently, 26 countries participate in the Visa Waiver

Pilot Program: Andorra, Argentina, Australia, Austria, Belgium, Brunei, Denmark, Finland, France, Germany, Iceland, Ireland, Italy, Japan, Lichtenstein, Luxembourg, Monaco, the Netherlands, New Zealand, Norway, San Marino, Slovenia, Spain, Sweden, Switzerland, and the United Kingdom. Visitors entering on the Visa Waiver Pilot Program cannot work or study while in the United States and cannot stay longer than 90 days or change their status to another category. If eligible, you may be able to avoid a trip to the U.S. consulate and avoid paying a fee. I strongly recommend that you make sure that you are eligible for this visa before getting on a plane, because even for citizens from the above-mentioned countries, some restrictions apply. Moreover, this visa has some specific limitations.

Do I Have to Stand in Line Outside the U.S. Consulate to Apply for the Visa?

You may not have to. Some U.S. consulates have drop-box facilities for certain eligible applicants. That means you can just drop the required documents in the box and collect the visa at the designated time. Ask your local U.S. consulate if you qualify.

J-1/J-2 VISA

The J-1 is the visa used by IMGs to be able to perform service as a member of the medical profession or to receive graduate medical education in the United States. Under the provision of Public Law 94-484, certain alien physicians are required to pass parts 1 and 2 of the National Board of Medical Examiners (NBME) or an equivalent examination before they can perform services as members of the medical profession. The Secretary of Health and Human Services has recognized USMLE steps 1 and 2 and the FMGEMS as the equivalent of NBME 1 and 2. The J visa is for educational and cultural exchange programs designated by the U.S. Information Agency (USIA). USIA has designated ECFMG to sponsor foreign national physicians as J-1 exchange visitors for participation in accredited programs of graduate medical education in the United States. The objectives of this program are to enhance international exchange in the field of medicine and promote mutual understanding between the people of the United States and those in other countries through the exchange of persons, knowledge, and skills.

Basic Requirements for a J-1 Visa

First, the applicant should have passed USMLE 1 and 2 or the former VQE (visa qualifying exam) or FMGEMS. Although VQE and FMGEMS have been slowly phased out, this is a relatively recent change and some IMGs may have taken different tests in combination. For example, some people have taken USMLE 1 and FMGEMS 2 or various other combinations. You can get in touch with ECFMG to determine if your combination qualifies you for J-1 and for USMLE 3. USMLE 3 has to be successfully taken before applying for a license in any state in the United States. It is important to understand completely the eligibility obtained with your combination of exams. A few of my colleagues in residency got into the residency on the basis of FMGEMS but then had to take USMLE 1, 2, and 3 before being eligible to apply for a license in any state in the United States.

Second, the applicant should have a valid standard ECFMG certificate. I want to emphasize the term *valid* here. The ECFMG certificate is valid for 2 years after you have passed USMLE 1 and 2 and the ECFMG English test or TOEFL (Test of English as a Foreign Language). Once you enter an accredited residency program, you are eligible to have your certificate permanently validated. If you do not enter a residency program right after taking the exams, keep the expiration date on your certificate in mind so that you do not find yourself with a residency prospect and no valid ECFMG certificate. If your ECFMG certificate expires, you will have to retake TOEFL. (TOEFL replaced the ECFMG English test as of March 3, 1999.) Expiration of the ECFMG certificate also applies to the CSA. If you have not entered a residency program within three years of passing the CSA, you will have to retake the exam.

Third, the applicant should hold a contract or letter of offer for a position in the accredited program.

Fourth, the applicant should provide a letter from the ministry of health in the country of nationality or of last legal residence. This is a written assurance by the home country that they need specialists in the area in which the exchange visitor will receive training in the United States. ECFMG provides you with the format of the letter. The organization insists on the exact language as stated in the form letter. You will have to ask the office of the ministry of health in your country about the office that deals with these letters. The same office also publishes the list of specializations that your country needs. This list differs for different countries, and you will have to see if the field of your training is included in that list. However, this requirement does not seem to be a big problem for people who want to apply for J-1 visa.

After you sign a contract for residency with a program, you will be sent an application package. Once the application process is complete, you will receive an IAP-66 form from your residency program. You then need to go to the embassy in your country to apply for the visa.

The application process is just like that for a tourist visa. You have to fill out form OF-156, which can be obtained at any U.S. consulate free of charge or downloaded from the Internet at *travel.state.gov/visa_services.html*. This simple form can be filled out on the day of your visit to the embassy. You need to bring your IAP-66 form, a valid passport, a photograph, a nonrefundable fee, and a visa fee if applicable. Once again, you have to demonstrate that you have ties that will attract you back to your country. No one can specify what form these ties could take. A few IMGs I have talked to suggest the following as examples that prove your bond to the home country:

- Your family ties: Mention close family such as parents, brothers, and sisters who live in the home country.
- Your professional ties. For example, if you are working in a well-known institute, doing an important work in your field, making a lot of money, say so.
- Your financial ties. If you belong to a very rich family, it is worth mentioning. It is a good idea to have the proof of ownership of a house or other property.
- Your community ties. If you have had a long association with a local organization and have done a considerable amount of work for it, you should mention it.

Visa Application

If you enter the United States on a J-1 visa, you have the obligation to return to the country of last residence for a specified period before you can change it to a work visa. If your ultimate aim is to try to practice in the United States, try to enter on an H-1 visa.

You should apply for the J-1 visa at the U.S. embassy or consulate with jurisdiction over your place of permanent residence. This is not always possible. For instance, some IMGs come to the United States on a tourist or student visa. Once there, they then try to secure residency and convert their original visa to a J-1. In this case, the IMG has to apply for the visa at the U.S. embassy in Mexico or Canada. If you are in this situation, it may be more difficult, though not impossible to qualify for this visa from outside your country of permanent residence.

Furthermore, you will be viewed with suspicion because you told a different story when you came to the United States the first time. In the case of a tourist visa, you would have stated that you were coming to the United States for interviews or (worse) pleasure. Now that you are not doing what you initially said, your intentions will become suspect. For these reasons, it is recommended that such individuals return to their home countries to apply for the J-1 visa; however, many IMGs are afraid they will be refused the visa in the home country and will never be able to reenter the United States.

Family Members

The dependents of a person with a J-1 visa can enter the United States on a dependent visa, called a J-2 visa. If you include the names of your dependents on the paperwork for the J-1, those names should appear on the IAP-66. Your family can apply for the visa at the same time you do or do it later by presenting your IAP to the counselor.

Some people suggest that you should tell the counselor you are not going to take your family to the United States. Their logic is that if you say to the counselor that you are going to the United States with your wife and child, it may make them think that you plan to settle permanetly in the United States. People sitting in the consulate think at a very realistic and human level. If you try to tell them that you are going to leave your family behind for 3 to 7 years, you are likely to come across as a very dishonest person.

The adult dependents of a person with a J-1 (J-2) can easily get permission to work.

Can a Person with a J-2 Work?

Your spouse with a J-2 can get a permit to work by applying to the INS. It is a very simple procedure. Call the INS office for the latest information about the paperwork needed. Apart from items that must be supplied to obtain the permit, you need to show proof that the money that your dependent spouse (J-2) is going to make by working is not meant to help you (J-1) support your family. This proof can take the form of a simple letter with two columns. In one column, list your monthly expenses, including expenses for lodging, car payment, gas, house utilities (including electricity, water, and phone) and so forth. In the other column, list your (J-1) monthly salary. The expenses should be less than the salary. This shows that your (J-1) salary is enough to support your family. As a proof of salary, you should attach your paystub. The

J-2 spouse must attach a letter explaining how he or she intends to use the additional money. This can be anything from going to school to going around the world. It is fairly easy to get the work permit, and a J-2 person with a work permit can do practically any job.

U.S. Port of Entry

As mentioned earlier, a visa does not guarantee entry into the United States. The INS has authority to deny admission. At the port of entry, an INS official validates Form I-94, Record of Arrival-Departure, which notes the length of stay permitted. Sometimes the form is marked D/S, which means your visa is valid for "duration of stay." But you still need to have a valid IAP-66 at all times. As long as you have an IAP-66 that is valid on a given date, you have legal status in the United States even if the visa stamped on your passport has expired.

Applying for the New IAP

If you enter a residency program in the United States, your contract with that program will be valid for 1 year with the understanding that it will be renewed every year. The renewal is based on your satisfactory performance in the program or continued liking of the program. An IAP is issued for 1 year at a time, and so you have to apply for a new IAP-66 every year. That means more paperwork and another source of anxiety. Usually ECFMG sends out the application forms for new IAPs about 4 months in advance to physicians in training who have a J-1 visa. The form needs to be filled out and sent back along with the required documents within a reasonable time to ensure that you receive your new IAP before the old one expires. If you are not able to gather the required documents in time, it may become a big headache. The most time-consuming step is getting the letter from the ministry of health in your country. That needs to be done every year if the previously submitted letter was designated for 1 year. Table 2–4 provides several tips to help you through this process.

Limitations of the J-1 Visa

This is a great visa with a very pious mission. It is a very helpful instrument if you are interested in coming to the United States for a limited period to receive training in a particular field of medicine. But its

If you have to get a "no objection" letter from the health ministry in your country before applying for an IAP, work hard on getting it for the total duration of training, not just for 1 year.

TABLE 2–4. Tips for Obtaining a Letter from the Ministry of Health

1. Try to get a letter that is valid for the total duration of your residency. This is legal and possible, and it makes sense because you are obviously going to finish the residency, which lasts a minimum of 3 years. This letter is in a way permission from your country to leave the country for the training in the field permitted. It is appropriate that you get permission for the traditional duration of the training.
2. If you cannot do this, start the work required to obtain this letter well in advance because when you are away from your country, you may not have a lot of control over things back home.
3. Get the name of the appropriate officials in your country from the embassy of your country in the United States and try talking to them personally.
4. The most important part is knowing the fields of training in which your country requires specialists. It can be tricky formulating the language of request letter. For example, if you are doing a cardiology fellowship, you may get the letter from one country easily if you say that it will include training in interventional cardiology. To get the letter from another country, you may be better off saying that training will include electrophysiology. Actually, you will get training in all these fields in a good cardiology fellowship program.
5. If things are late in arriving from your country, apply for the letter at your country's embassy in the United States. Most countries authorize their consulates in the United States to issue at least time-bound letters. That should give you a lot of time to get the pending items from your country.

limitations can be bothersome if you are using the J-1 visa to get a foot in the door with the final mission of ultimately settling in the United States. Because the J-1 visa puts a cap on your total stay in the country, if you later want to apply for permanent residence, you must first return to the country of your permanent residence for a specified period (2 years at the time of the writing of this book). Lately, the U.S. government has taken a number of steps to discourage individuals with J-1 visas from staying in the United States. The main points I want to clarify for you are as follows:

- "Going back to your country" before applying for permanent status means that you have to return to the country that was your legal residence before you came to the United States. This means you cannot go to work in another country that might pay doctors more than your own country does.
- There is a way to avoid returning back to your country, popularly called "getting a waiver." This involves working at a place or for an organization that has been designated specifically for the

purpose of giving waiver jobs to J-1 holders. As an example, you might work in an area with a physician shortage or for a government organization. The responsibility for getting the job is yours. In all cases, you are required to work for a minimum period in the designated position before you can become eligible for permanent residence in the United States. At the time of writing this book, this period was 5 years, but it may change. If you are trying to enter a residency program in the United States with the intent of ultimately settling there, the J-1 visa probably is not the best choice. A better option may be the H-1 visa, discussed later in this chapter.

- You are supposed to hold employment and receive financial gain only from the position that you were given the visa for. This looks obvious, but it may not seem all right once you are in a residency program in the United States and are not eligible for moonlighting.

J-1 Research Visa

Some IMGs have come to the United States on a J-1 research visa with the aim of changing to a J-1 once they get into a residency position. The United States Information Agency has issued a compilation of existing policies which was published in the *Federal Register* on June 30, 1999, vol. 64, no. 125; pp. 34982–34983. Part of this statement states that IMGs cannot get sponsorship for graduate medical education if they have been research scholars or professor participants in the preceding 12 months.

Traveling on the J-1 Visa

There are no limitations on a person with a J-1 visa traveling outside the country, but you need to be aware of the documentation required before you leave the United States.

> If you want to travel on a J-1 visa, you need to apply for a new IAP-66 in addition to the one you already have. ECFMG advises that this should be done well in advance. Faxing your request to ECFMG can accomplish this. You do not need to have a visa stamped on your passport before leaving the United States, but you have to have it stamped on your passport before entering again.

This can be a worrisome issue because some IMGs may not have a visa stamped on their passports despite having a valid IAP-66. If you do not have a valid visa when you leave the United States, you can do one of two things:

1. You can leave and get the visa stamped at the port of arrival. However, some IMGs fear they may be refused the visa once they are in the home country. If this were to happen, they could not get back into the United States. If that is your concern, do the following.
2. You can go to a country with contiguous borders with the United States and get the visa stamped there. The procedure for doing that is explained later in this chapter.

H-1/H-4 VISA

The H-1 visa is called a temporary worker visa. As it applies to doctors, it means that you should have a residency position in hand when you apply. Your employer also must complete some paperwork. For this visa, you do not have to get any papers from ECFMG, unlike the J-1 visa. Here are some salient points:

You must have passed USMLE step 3 before you can apply for an H-1 visa for residency training.

- To be eligible for this visa, you must have cleared USMLE 3. This test should be taken in almost all situations. Some IMGs have been told by "lawyers" that they can do a residency on an H-1 visa without passing the USMLE 3, but I am not aware of any IMG succeeding in that.
- The H-1 is a good visa if you plan to stay in the United States. There is no obligation for an H-1 resident to return to the country of last legal residence, unlike the J-1. Even while you are doing a residency on this visa, you can try to apply for a green card. Most IMGs are unaware of such possibilities. Most people who do try to do it are green card holders by the end of the residency. All it takes is a good lawyer and good standing in your profession. Everybody who gets into a residency should start looking at these possibilities at the very beginning of the residency. Time is of the essence here because if your lawyer feels that you need to add some frills to your curriculum vitae before you become eligible for a green card petition, you may be able to work toward this goal as you proceed in the residency.

- There is a fixed quota for H-1 visas every year; this quota is decided for all professionals together. This means software engineers and people from other professions are sharing the pie with you. H-1 petitions are granted on merit, but the doors are closed once the quota is exhausted. The acceptance of applications starts in October. You should try to interview in September or October and see if there are institutions that offer a residency "out of match" (that is, not through the residency matching program). That way you can get your application in a little ahead of time. This is easier said than done because some programs may not start interviewing before October and most programs do not want to offer residency out of match, but you can always try.
- Once you have an H-1 visa, your dependents are able to obtain an H-4 visa. If you have a spouse who intends to work, he or she will have to arrange his or her own visa before being allowed to work. This can be important if your spouse is also a doctor. He or she will have to pass the USMLE 3 before starting a residency, which may not be easy. Sometimes H-4 spouses have to join a residency on a J-1. That defeats the purpose of working hard to get an H-1 in the first place.
- There is a limit on the total period you can stay in the United States on an H-1 visa. At the time of writing this book, it was 6 years.

If you are looking to do a residency on this visa, you should discuss this at the time of your interview. Some programs may not be willing to sponsor you for the H-1 visa. After you sign a contract with a residency program, the following steps have to be taken. The residency program usually does all the paperwork through its own lawyer. Most programs will foot the lawyer's bill, but some may insist that you pay the fee. The steps are as follows:

1. Obtain labor department permission. This step is designed to safeguard the interests of employees (in this case, you). The labor department wants to make sure that the stipend you get is equivalent to what others get for the same kind of work.
2. After this, your program will file an I-129 with the INS for approval. Once it is approved, you will receive a copy of the approval form, I-797. You can then go to the local embassy of your country with those papers to get the visa stamped.

Required Documentation

Each applicant for a temporary worker visa must pay a nonrefundable application fee (US$45 at the time of writing of this book) and submit the following:

1. An application form OF-156, completed and signed.
2. A passport valid for travel to the United States with a validity date at least 6 months beyond the applicant's intended period of stay. If more than one person is included in the passport, each person desiring a visa must make an application.
3. A 1 and 1/2 inch square (37 × 37 mm) photograph for each applicant, showing the full face against a light background.
4. A notice of approval, Form I-797. If you receive this approval while you are in the United States, you will have to go to Mexico or Canada to get the visa stamped on your passport. But as long as you have a valid I-797, you have legal status in the United States.

It often happens that an IMG is in the United States when he or she gets a J-1 or H-1 visa. You may not be ready to return to your country to get the visa stamped. In this case you may have to apply for the visa at a border post. The following text summarizes the information given by the Department of State about this process.

Applying for a Visa at a Border Post if You Are a Third World National in the United States

- **Appointments.** Any third country national (TCN) present in the United States and visitors present in Canada who wish to apply for a nonimmigrant visa at any border post in Canada or Mexico must make an appointment for an interview. U.S. Consular offices are located in Calgary, Halifax, Montreal, Ottawa, Quebec City, Toronto, Vancouver, Ciudad Juarez, Matamoros, and Tijuana.
- **Appointments by Telephone.** If you are in the United States and you wish to schedule an appointment, you should call 1-900-443-3131; in Canada you should call 1-900-451-2778 (*there is a high per minute charge for these calls*). Callers from the United States or Canada who wish to charge the cost of the call to a credit card may schedule an appointment by calling

1-888-840-0032. Unlike the 1-900 numbers, which are blocked from most hotels, office, or pay telephones, the credit card line can be accessed from virtually any telephone. The appointment system requires a touch-tone phone; a push-button rotary phone will not work.

- **Appointment by Internet.** Applicants can also book appointments via the Internet at *http://www.nvars.com* Each appointment costs $30 Canadian at the time of writing this book, which will be charged to a major credit card. Applicants are advised to have their credit card information handy. After your appointment is scheduled, you will be mailed an application form (OF-156) and an information sheet for the post where you will be applying. You should not call an individual post directly to request an appointment. These appointments can *only* be scheduled by calling the appropriate 1-900 or 1-888 telephone number or by using the Internet.

Who Can Be Issued a Visa at a Border Post?

- **Hours of Operation.** Operators are available from 7 A.M. to 10 P.M. Eastern Time. Callers may have difficulty getting through if they call during the peak times of 7 A.M., 11 A.M.,

Individuals who have ever been out of status in the United States because they overstayed their visa are not eligible to apply at a border post. In other words, if you have remained in the United States longer than the period authorized by the immigration officer when you entered the United States in any visa category, you must apply in the country of your nationality. If you are not certain about your status, check with the nearest INS office.

Individuals seeking appointments should be aware that applicants may be more likely to encounter difficulties at the time of interview when they apply for a visa outside of their home country. Consular officers at border posts will deny visas whenever they believe there are fraud indicators present, or their lack of knowledge of local conditions and familiarity with documents in the applicant's home country prevents them from properly adjudicating the case.

None of the border posts will accept applications for E visas from TCN applicants who are not resident in their consular districts.

2 P.M., 4:30 P.M., and 7 P.M. Eastern Time. Appointments for border posts outside the Eastern Time Zone can only be made after it is 7 A.M. in the post's time zone. The Internet system is available 24 hours a day, seven days a week.

- **Additional Information.** Applicants who are unable to attend their scheduled appointments must cancel them 2 full working days prior to the appointment by calling toll-free 1-888-611-6676. Would-be applicants who do not need a visa to remain in the United States may find it more convenient to apply for a visa elsewhere in conjunction with their next foreign travel. Those who plan to visit Canada, Mexico, or, in the cases of students and exchange visitors, adjacent islands, may reenter the United States within 30 days on expired visas as long as they possess a valid I-94 form. Visa applicants should take their appointment letters to the interview. They may be admitted without one, but absence of the letter could cause delays. Certain nationalities require visas from Canadian authorities in order to enter Canada.

IMMIGRATION

You can come to the United States as an immigrant on the following bases:

- You have a blood relation who is eligible to sponsor you. The details of this route are beyond the scope of this book.
- You marry someone who is a U.S. citizen.

Doctors from the same ethnic group are a desirable commodity for people settled in the United States, who have children of marriageable age. Frequently, parents who are first-generation Americans think that children from their country of origin have stronger family values and have a stronger character. In addition, doctors from the home country have the potential to earn a good living once they are in the United States. The parents may also be anxious about the possibility of their children marrying someone from a different ethnic group. All of these factors lead first-generation parents to look for marriageable men or women from their country of origin, and people in the medical profession are a popular choice. This is a symbiotic relationship, and many IMGs have come to the United States on the basis of marriage. This action has the potential to provide stable visa status if you are bent on staying in the United States.

If you are coming to the United States on the basis of marrying a U.S. citizen, be sure you know that person well. When you first arrive, you will probably be so excited about getting into the country that no sacrifice will seem too great. I have seen people who arrived in the United States after meeting their prospective wife or husband only once or twice or not meeting them at all. In some unfortunate situations, their relationship problems began as soon as they landed at the airport. This can be a heartbreaking experience. Often these new immigrants do not want to return to their country of origin, and they try to rough it out here. It may be many years before they are able to resolve these problems. Unfortunately, numerous examples of this situation can be found in the United States.

Carefully evaluate your options before jumping on the first proposition that can get you to the United States.

Most IMGs who enter the United States through this route are relatively young. These are the people who are the most likely to lose focus on their real goal. Keep in mind, it can be very painful to be dependent on your spouse for every penny. This will be the situation while you are preparing for exams after coming to the U.S. For this reason, I strongly suggest you pass the USMLE 1 and 2 exams before coming to this country. You should do that even if you have to postpone your trip for a year or two. It may be frustrating, but this is what you need to do if you want things to go smoothly once you are in America. Even if you are coming to the United States on an immigrant visa, you should plan your itinerary similar to that of someone planning to come here on a J-1 visa. By that I mean, again, you should have passed these exams before coming here. Discussions with numerous IMGs have revealed that it is much easier to pass the USMLE exams in your own country. The main reasons for this are the presence of greater emotional support, and the awareness that you have other options even if you do not pass the exams. That takes away a lot of the anxiety associated with taking the exams.

ABOUT FORM OF-156

I mentioned Form OF-156 earlier in this chapter. This form must be filled out practically every time you go to the U.S. embassy, and it can be filled out the day you go to apply for the visa. While it is a very simple form, the fear of the unknown and the fear of writing something wrong sometimes makes people very nervous. Table 2–5 reproduces Form OF-156. Tips on filling out the form are presented in Table 2–6.

TABLE 2-5. Tips on Completing Form OF-156

1. SURNAMES OR FAMILY NAMES *(Exactly as in Passport)*

2. FIRST NAME AND MIDDLE NAME *(Exactly as in Passport)*

3. OTHER NAMES *(Maiden, Religious, Professional Aliases)*

4. DATE OF BIRTH *(Day, Month, Year)*

8. PASSPORT NUMBER

5. PLACE OF BIRTH
City, Province   Country

DATE PASSPORT ISSUED *(Day, Month, Year)*

DATE PASSPORT EXPIRES *(Day, Month, Year)*

6. NATIONALITY

7. SEX
☐ MALE
☐ FEMALE

9. HOME ADDRESS *(Include apartment No., street, city, province and postal zone)*

10. NAME AND ADDRESS OF PRESENT EMPLOYER OR SCHOOL
(Postal box number unacceptable)

11. HOME TELEPHONE NO.

12. BUSINESS TELEPHONE NO.

13. MARITAL STATUS
☐ Married ☐ Single ☐ Widowed ☐ Divorced ☐ Separated
If married, give name and nationality of spouse

14. NAMES AND RELATIONSHIPS OF PERSONS TRAVELING WITH YOU
(NOTE: A separate application must be made for a visa for each traveler, regardless of age.)

15. HAVE YOU EVER APPLIED FOR A U.S. VISA?
☐ No ☐ Yes
TYPE OF VISA? ____
WHERE? ____
WHEN? ____
☐ Visa was issued ☐ Visa was refused

16. HAS YOUR U.S. VISA EVER BEEN CANCELLED?
☐ No ☐ Yes
WHERE? ____
WHEN? ____
BY WHOM? ____

37 mm X 37 mm
PHOTO
GLUE PHOTO HERE

FORM 0F-156Y (VAC 2/99)

17. Bearers of visitors visas may generally not work or study in the U.S.
DO YOU INTEND TO WORK IN THE U.S.? ☐ No ☐ Yes
If YES, explain.

18. DO YOU INTEND TO STUDY IN THE U.S.? ☐ No ☐ Yes
(If YES, write name and address of school as it appears on form I-20)

19. PRESENT OCCUPATION *(If retired, state past occupation)*

20. WHO WILL FURNISH FINANCIAL SUPPORT, INCLUDING TICKETS?

21. AT WHAT ADDRESS WILL YOU STAY IN THE U.S.A.?

22. WHAT IS THE PURPOSE OF YOUR TRIP?

23. WHEN DO YOU INTEND TO ARRIVE IN THE U.S.A.?

24. HOW LONG DO YOU PLAN TO STAY IN THE U.S.A.?

25. HAVE YOU EVER BEEN IN THE U.S.A.?
☐ No ☐ Yes
WHEN? ____
HOW LONG? ____

26. HAVE YOU OR ANYONE ACTING FOR YOU EVER INDICATED TO A U.S. CONSULAR OR IMMIGRATION EMPLOYEE A DESIRE TO IMMIGRATE TO THE U.S. OR HAVE YOU EVER ENTERED A U.S. VISA LOTTERY?
☐ No ☐ Yes
HAS ANYONE EVER FILED AN IMMIGRANT VISA PETITION ON YOUR BEHALF?
☐ No ☐ Yes
HAS A LABOR CERTIFICATION FOR EMPLOYMENT IN THE U.S. EVER BEEN REQUESTED BY YOU OR ON YOUR BEHALF?
☐ No ☐ Yes

27. ARE ANY OF THE FOLLOWING IN THE U.S., RESIDE IN THE US., OR HAVE U.S. LEGAL PERMANENT RESIDENCE?
(Circle YES or NO and indicate that person's status in the U.S., i.e. studying, working, permanent resident, U.S. citizen, etc.)

YES NO Husband/Wife ____ YES NO Fiance/Fiancee ____ YES NO Brother/Sister ____

YES NO Father/Mother ____ YES NO Son/Daughter ____

28. WHERE HAVE YOU LIVED FOR THE PAST FIVE YEARS? DO NOT INCLUDE PLACES YOU HAVE VISITED FOR PERIODS OF SIX MONTHS OR LESS.
Countries   Cities   Approximate Dates

29. IMPORTANT: ALL APPLICANTS MUST READ AND CHECK THE APPROPRIATE BOX FOR EACH ITEM:

A visa may not be issued to persons who are within specific categories defined by law as inadmissible to the United States (except when a waiver is obtained in advance). Are any of the following applicable to you?

- Have you ever been afflicted with a communicable disease of public health significance, a dangerous physical or mental disorder, or been a drug abuser or addict?[212(a)(1)] ☐ Yes ☐ No
- Have you ever been arrested or convicted for any offense or crime, even though subject of a pardon, amnesty or other similar legal action? Have you ever lawfully distributed or sold a controlled substance (drug), or been a prostitute or procurer for prositiutes?[212(a)(2)] ☐ Yes ☐ No
- Do you seek to enter the United States to engage in export control violations, subversive or terrorist activities, or any other unlawful purpose? Are you a member or representative fo a terrorist organization as currently designated by the U.S. Secretary of State? Have you ever participated in persecutions directed by the Nazi government of Germany, or have you ever participated in genocide?[212(a)(3)] ☐ Yes ☐ No
- Have you ever been refused admission to the U.S., or the subject of a deportation hearing, or sought to obtain a visa or any U.S. Immigration benefit by fraud or wilful misrepresentation? Have you attended a U.S. public elementary school on student(F) status, or a public secondary school without reimbursing the school after November 30, 1996? [212(a)(6)] ☐ Yes ☐ No
- Have you ever departed or remained outside the United States to avoid military service? [212(a)(8)] ☐ Yes ☐ No
- Have you ever violated the terms of a U.S. visa, or been unlawfully present in, or deported from the U.S.A.? [212(a)(9)] ☐ Yes ☐ No
- Have you ever withheld custody of a U.S. citizen child, outside the United States from a person granted legal custody by a U.S. court, voted in the United States in violation of any law or regulation, or renounced U.S. citizenship for the purpose of avoiding taxation? [212(a)(10)] ☐ Yes ☐ No

A YES answer does not automatically signify ineligibility for a visa, but if you answered YES to any of the above, or if you have any question in this regard, personal appearance at this office is recommended. If appearance is not possible at this time, attach a statement of facts in your case to the application.

30. I certify that I have read and understood all the questions set forth in this application and the answers I have furnished on this form are true and correct to the best of my knowledge and belief. I understand that any false or misleading statement may result in the permanent refusal of visa or denial of entry into the United States. I understand that possession of a visa does not entitle the bearer to enter the United States of America upon arrival at port of entry if he or she is found inadmissible.

DATE OF APPLICATION ____

APPLICANT'S SIGNATURE ____
If this application has been prepared by a travel agency or another person on your behalf, the agent should indicate name and address of agency or person with appropriate signature of individual preparing form.

SIGNATURE OF PERSON PREPARING FORM ____
(If other than applicant)

DO NOT WRITE IN THIS SPACE

B-1 / B-2 MAX   B-1 MAX   B-2 MAX   ISSUED   214(b)   221(g)

OTHER ____ MAX   ON ____ BY ____
Visa Classification

MULTI OR ____   OTHER ____
Number Applications

MONTHS ____   REFUSAL REVIEWED BY ____
Validity

THIS FORM MAY NOT BE ACCEPTED AT ALL CONSULATES OR EMBASSIES.

Table 2–6. **Tips on Completing Form OF-156**

1–14	Baseline info.
15 & 16.	Give them the facts, understanding that they may have the information about your previous attempts in their computer anyway.
17.	At the time of applying for B-1 visa, say no. When you are applying for J-1, say yes.
18.	Working on J-1 or going for CSA or for interviews is not exactly studying.
19.	You should try to explain your occupation in the best possible manner. A good job may be seen as one of the incentives for you to return to your country after training in the United States. (Remember the requirements for getting the J-1 or H-1 visa?)
20.	It is better to say 'yourself' if you have worked in your country for a while. This also shows your firm position in your country.
21.	If you are not sure, say you will look around and stay in a hotel or motel.
22.	Tell the truth.
23.	Tell the approximate month.
24.	Tell the approximate time (preferably at least 3 months) for B-1 visa and 3–7 years for J-1 visa.
25 & 26.	Tell the truth.
27.	I would not necessarily try to dig up a distant relative or a cursory acquaintance just to put some name there. After all, each name appearing in this column is a potential attraction that may be likely to keep you back in the United States.
28 & 29.	This is some information about yourself.

CHAPTER 3

Preparing for the Exams

WHO NEEDS TO TAKE THE EXAMS?

Any doctor who expects to work in a position that involves direct patient care or whose decisions will directly affect patients in the United States must pass the USMLE steps 1 and 2, the CSA, and the English examination. This applies to those planning to enter all clinical fields, including radiology and pathology. You may not have to take these exams if you plan to do bench research or research that involves working only on animals.

> IMGs are sometimes advised that persons who plan to pursue careers in pharmacology or microbiology do not have to pass the USMLE exams. In some countries, candidates train in these fields after having attained a medical degree and a license for practicing medicine in their countries. Such positions may not have similar counterparts in the United States. For example, in the United States, a person does not have to graduate from medical school before pursuing a career in microbiology. If you are a foreign medical doctor with special training in microbiology and have not passed the USMLE, the highest position you will probably achieve in the United States is that of a supervisor in a microbiology laboratory. My wife found herself in a similar situation, and we learned this simple piece of information only after a lot of research. It may be true for other basic fields as well. I would suggest you research this before you come to the United States.

Anyone who wants to practice clinical medicine in any form must be ECFMG certified by taking and passing exams.

IMGs are trained at different institutions around the world, and these institutions have their own strengths and weaknesses. The USMLE exams are designed to ensure a baseline level of knowledge and a doctor's ability to apply that knowledge to actual patient care.

The baseline is that body of knowledge judged to be sufficient for the proper care of patients.

In later chapters, I will provide tips to help you do well on the specific exams and later, in your residency program. Many books and coaching courses are available that are designed to prepare medical graduates to take the exams. Often, IMGs are not aware of the resources and strategies that can help *them* in their preparations. In addition, most IMG examinees face several inherent obstacles when preparing to take the exams, as detailed in Table 3–1. This chapter provides strategies to help you overcome these obstacles.

TABLE 3–1. Obstacles Facing IMG Examinees

1. Most IMGs are motivated to study hard, but sometimes they do not know the books that will help them prepare well for the exams. Choose a good board review book; if you are not sure which book to choose, discuss it with your friends.
2. Most IMGs do not know what they need to know to do well on the exams. This is because they learned medicine in a way that enabled them to do well in medical school and to treat patients in their country well. However, this may not equate with the approach to medicine in the exams.
3. Most IMGs who fall into the painful rut of failing the exams multiple times are not aware of what I call the "soul of the exam." A real-life story deserves mention here. It is the story of a friend of mine whom I know to be a very intelligent person and a good doctor. He notes: "I took the USMLE 1 and failed miserably. I studied again with greater vigor only to fail again. One failure led to another. My parents came from India to see me and suggested that I should settle for a technician's job. Their comments hurt me a lot. The memories of my glorious medical career in India haunted me constantly. I read my books continuously to the extent that I could flip through the whole of a biochemistry book in less than an hour. I still failed. Then someone coached me on what is expected of the examinees in these exams. I passed with flying colors the very next time. I think the only thing I lacked all those years was the knowledge of the soul of this exam." Today, this friend of mine is doing very well in his residency.
4. Most IMGs have little idea of how medicine is actually practiced in the United States. Because IMGs do not know what is expected of a physician in the United States, it is difficult for them to do well on the exams.
5. For some IMGs, the USMLE may be the first exam that exposes them to this particular style of questions. IMGs may have been required to write essay-type answers for exams throughout their lives. Review books that contain practice exams with USMLE-type questions can provide the experience needed to surmount this problem.

GENERAL INFORMATION

Armed with the knowledge I have gained from interviewing numerous IMGs, I have designed this chapter to help you prepare confidently for the exams. First off, you need to remember that to reach the current point in your academic career, you must have already done very well in the numerous exams for which you have prepared. Only a well-motivated person and a good exam taker can get into and make it out of medical school successfully. A physician's life is a series of exams. These latest exams are simply the next steps in your career.

I do not think that I should be telling you what to eat before you take the USMLE. Do whatever has worked for you all these years. If you think a particular color brings you good luck, wear it. If the lucky bracelet around your wrist has worked for you so far, keep it on. Remember, the USMLE is just another exam. Eight things the exam is *not* are presented in Table 3–2.

COMPUTER-BASED TESTING

Computer-based testing (CBT) is the new method of testing for the USMLE. Examinees will now take the examination on the computer as opposed to reading questions from and marking answers on a piece of paper.

CBT, as opposed to a pencil-and-paper exam, has several advantages:

- It offers greater examination security.
- It permits new assessment methods to be used.
- It allows increased flexibility in scheduling.

The main advantage of the computer test will be that you can take the USMLE at any time of the year. This removes the pressure on IMGs to appear for an exam on a preset date.

THE SYLVAN CENTER

This is a chain of centers that administers tests on behalf of various agencies. The tests that they give include the TOEFL and GRE. They have centers in different countries throughout the world. This same agency has been selected by USMLE to give steps 1 and 2 of the test throughout the world.

To do well on the exams, you need to think like a doctor practicing in the United States.

TABLE 3–2. What the USMLE Is Not

1. It is not like some professors' clinical rounds where you are tested about esoteric and rare entities.
2. It is not checking your memory/recall (e.g., by answering questions such as "what is Noonan's syndrome?").
3. It is not designed to test a narrow range of knowledge. You cannot do well by mastering a few topics. As you know, you have to answer about 800 questions for each step. The examiners have the opportunity to test you on every subject. This situation is unlike that in some countries where examinees can concentrate on only those topics they have come to know are important over the course of their classroom teaching.
4. It is not designed with your background in mind. You are at a slight disadvantage as compared to U.S. graduates who were taught by teachers with a full grasp of the format of the board exams. Your medical school professor did not design this test. Thus, you may be less prepared to prioritize your study of the topics covered.
5. It is not representative of the country where you trained for your medical degree. Medical exams in different countries will differ in the importance they place on various disease processes, depending on the prevalence of those disease processes in the local community. You need to remember that for the purposes of the USMLE, you are supposed to have more knowledge about diseases that are more prevalent in the United States. This often requires thorough study of diseases that may be nonexistent in your country of origin. In later chapters I will touch on the topics that you must cover. These are topics that IMGs are likely to ignore.
6. It is not testing your knowledge of the most expensive test available for the diagnosis of a given disease. IMGs often suppose that every patient with a headache is sent for magnetic resonance imaging (MRI) and every person with vomiting undergoes endoscopy in the United States. This stems from the knowledge that the United States is a technologically advanced country. Just because technology is available, however, it is not used offhandedly. The examiners want to be sure you will manage a patient in the most cost-effective and efficient way. That means you have to give due credit to the history and physical exam and simple laboratory tests. You also have to act on the basis of the pretest probability before ordering a test and have to see if the result of that test is likely to have any bearing on your management decisions.
7. It is not a test of your management decisions using the techniques available in your home country. Some tests that are ordered infrequently in your country may be common in the United States. You need to be aware of such diagnostic or therapeutic modalities, and you should also know how to interpret such tests.
8. It is not easy.

Concerns and Suggested Solutions Regarding CBT

The ambience of this test will be very different from those you have taken before. Here, you will be sitting in a cubicle all by yourself with a computer. This is likely to take away one essential component that we have come to associate with exam-taking ever since childhood—anxiety. IMGs should practice answering test questions on the computer to gain familiarity with this ambience.

You must gain experience with computers before taking the examination. Do not depend on pretest tutorial.

Another concern is the computer naïveté of test takers. Computers today are very user friendly and, while taking a test on the computer does not require you to be a computer whiz, I know from personal experience as well as the experience of many others that one's first encounter with a computer always involves some degree of nervousness. It is like giving an intramuscular injection for the first time—a situation that makes medical students nervous even though those teaching the skill firmly believe the students' trepidation is an overreaction. Although the Sylvan centers will be offering tutorials immediately before the exam, IMGs will be at a disadvantage if the first time they work on a computer is at the exam center, pre-exam tutorial or no tutorial.

As a solution, the Sylvan centers will be providing practice sessions in the simulated ambience for an extra fee. I expect that some entrepreneurial students in other countries may go into business coaching prospective examinees in an introductory session with the computers, to simulate the real exam. I strongly recommend that you take advantage of such opportunities to gain experience with the computers before sitting for the exam.

REGISTRATION

You will have to write to ECFMG for application forms and instructional materials. Once you complete the form and send it to the ECFMG, your eligibility for the exam will be confirmed. You will then be sent authorization of your eligibility and instructions for making an appointment at a test center. Your eligibility authorization will specify the 90-day period during which you will have to complete the exam. Because the dates for the exam are allotted on a first-come, first-served basis, you may not be able to get an appointment at the time you want it. I would strongly urge you to call the exam center of your choice as soon as you receive the eligibility authorization.

RESCHEDULING THE EXAM

If you cannot take the exam on the scheduled date, you can cancel your appointment. There will be no charges for rescheduling as long as you make the change at least 2 days before the scheduled date. However, you still have to take the exam within the original 90-day eligibility period. Otherwise, you will have to apply all over again.

REEXAMINATION

In the unfortunate event that an examinee fails the exam, he or she must reapply with a new application and fee. An examinee can retake the same step after 60 days, and he or she can repeat the same step no more than three times in 12 months.

TAKING THE EXAM

WHERE TO TAKE THE TEST

While the CSA and USMLE 3 must be taken in the United States, IMGs are able to take the other required exams in several locations around the world. Many IMGs are not able to decide where they should go to take these tests. This decision is more difficult for those who become eligible to come to the United States for some reason, such as getting a green card. Often, these people are lured to come to the United States as soon as possible, sometimes before passing the USMLE 1 and 2. They may think they will be able to do better on the exams while in the United States. My research suggests the contrary—that it is easier to pass the exams as well as deal with a failure while in your own country. It is true that extra information is likely to be available in the United States. However, the chapters in this book should give you insight into the typical residency program in a United States hospital. Whenever possible, then, I recommend taking your exams before coming to the United States.

If a USMLE center is not located in your country, choose a center on the basis of following aspects:

- The cost of travel to the center
- The cost of boarding and lodging

- The similarity of the host country's food to that of your own country. I'm not kidding! Bad food can become a distracter during your preparation for the exams.

DRESSING FOR THE EXAM

Most of the exam centers are air-conditioned, and the temperature set for the air conditioner may be too cold for some examinees. You may feel chilly sitting still in the examination hall. Be sure to carry a thin sweater to the examination hall even if it is hot outside.

ON THE DAY OF THE EXAM

You will be expected to show an identification document (ID) with your photo and signature on it. For most IMGs, a passport will satisfy this requirement. You are expected to be on time. The USMLE bulletin states that if you are more than 30 minutes late, you will not be allowed to sit for the exam and you will have to register for the exam again.

When you arrive at the center on the day of the exam, your ID will be checked and your photo will be taken. You will be given a locker in which to place your personal belongings. Next, you will be given instructions about the computer equipment and the opportunity to complete a brief tutorial. After this, you will be ready to go under the vigilant eyes of the human as well as video monitors.

TIME MANAGEMENT DURING THE EXAM

You will be given questions in blocks of 30 and 60 minutes. If you leave the exam area for a break during a block of questions, your time will keep running and your departure from the exam area will be noted as an irregular incident (not behavior). For these reasons, you should avoid leaving the test area during a block. However, if you must leave for some reason, do not become excessively worried about it. These events are noted as irregular incidents to prevent unscrupulous examinees from gaining an unfair advantage (e.g., by engaging in unfair practices). If you are honest, you have no reason to worry.

You will be allowed time for breaks inbetween the blocks. Each candidate is allowed a total of 45 minutes per exam day for breaks, including time for lunch. You should use the breaks wisely. If you happen to finish some blocks before the time is up, the extra time will be yours for breaks.

Eat carefully during lunch or other breaks. Do not eat fatty foods or drink any beverages that might make you jittery or woozy. This simple caution can become a big challenge if you are traveling to another country to take the test. You may have no idea about the character of the food items available during lunchtime. For example, coffee available in the United States is likely to be much stronger than that available on the Indian subcontinent. Those innocent-looking American cookies could be loaded with fat. It is probably safest to stick to fruit, yogurt, or noncaffeinated beverages during the breaks.

Understand the aim and soul of the examination before you start with the review books.

UNDERSTANDING THE SOUL OF THE EXAMINATION

I think there is no better way to understand what I call the "soul of the exam" than to review several points covered in the book that is a resource for test item writers (Case SM, Swanson DB (1998) Constructing Written Test Questions for the Basic and Clinical Sciences, National Board of Medical Examiners®, 2nd ed.). (Available http://www.nbme.org/new.version/98.1.w.pdf)[1999, Dec. 14] This is one of the suggested readings for the examiners who write the test questions for the USMLE exams. Knowledge of how the questions are constructed and the intent behind the questions is invaluable for preparation for these exams. You should keep the following points in mind:

1. Through the questions asked, the examiners are trying to communicate what they view as important to the practice of medicine in the United States. This is meant to fill any instructional gaps by encouraging students to read broadly on their own, as well as to compensate for educational experiences that may vary from student to student. This is particularly true for IMGs who are trained in different institutions, and sometimes in different languages.
2. The test time devoted to each area is directly proportional to its importance in practical life.
3. People who write test questions for the USMLE are given suggestions on ways to avoid flaws that are likely to help test-wise students identify the desired answer. I suggest you avoid putting too much energy into finding the flaws, at the expense of "problem-solving" the questions. However, if you do not have a clue about a question, you may be able to gain some cues from technical flaws in the formulation of the question or its answer choices.

- Grammatical cues—The answer that does not fit grammatically with the question can be thrown out as wrong.
- Absolute terms—Some people think that choices using the words "never" or "always" are likely to be wrong.
- Length—The correct answer is likely to be long.
- Convergence strategy—The correct answer often has the most elements in common with other options. The reference referred to earlier states that this happens because item writers start with the correct answer and write permutations of this answer as the distracters. (Distracters are the incorrect choices that are presented as possible answers to a given question.)
- The middle ground—In case of numerical answers, the number that falls in the middle range is more likely to be correct than more extreme numbers.

4. The examiners do not waste time testing trivial facts.
5. They try to focus on an important concept or a potentially catastrophic clinical problem.
6. They try to avoid testing on esoteric or interesting topics, the knowledge of which is not essential for the practice of medicine.
7. Common misconceptions and faulty reasoning are usually chosen as distracters.
8. Application of knowledge is tested by using clinical vignettes to evaluate medical decision making in patient care situations.
9. Clinical situations that would be handled by a subspecialist are avoided.

LONG VIGNETTES: A METHOD TO THE MADNESS

Some IMGs I have interviewed felt that the time allocated to complete the test was too short. This problem is faced more commonly by IMGs from the countries where the medium of teaching medicine is other than English. These graduates tend to have more difficulty because most of the questions on the USMLE exams are in the form of half-page-long vignettes. These vignettes are often difficult to understand and very time-consuming to read. One solution is to practice answering similar questions in a testlike situation with a timer. This approach should help increase your reading speed. Another concern is that a long vignette often looks like a block of randomly strewn information. The common format of a vignette is as follows:

Age
Gender
Chief complaint
Site of care
Personal history
Physical examination
+/− results of diagnostic tests
+/− initial treatment
Subsequent findings

Awareness of this sequence will help you know what to look for as you read through the vignette.

A FEW LAST THINGS TO REMEMBER

Table 3–3 lists five tips to keep in mind while you are taking the exams.

TABLE 3–3. Five Things to Remember During the Exam

1. Deal with one question at a time. Answer the question in the best possible manner and move on. Do not leave questions intending to come back to them later. That approach can be very time consuming.
2. When reading long vignettes, read them carefully, the first time. Then attempt to answer the questions on the basis of all the information provided. These vignettes are no different from the case presentations you have had experience with in your countries.
3. Do not panic if you do not know the answers to several questions in a row. You are not the only person this is happening to. When you answer the question on the basis of an informed guess, you are likely to be right in many cases.
4. Keep an eye on the time, but do not try to rush through either.
5. Curb the tendency to change your answers if you have some time at the end of a block.

CHAPTER 4

USMLE Step 1

ELIGIBILITY CRITERIA FOR STEP 1

To be eligible to take the USMLE step 1, you should be a graduate of or a medical student officially enrolled in a medical school listed in the current edition of the *World Directory of Medical Schools*. If you are attending a foreign medical school at the time you enroll for the exam, you should have completed the basic science component of the medical school curriculum. This can correspond to different numbers of years of medical school in different countries.

WHAT IS THE WHO *WORLD DIRECTORY OF MEDICAL SCHOOLS*?

The World Health Organization (WHO) publishes the *World Directory of Medical Schools*. However, the organization has no authority to grant any form of recognition or accreditation to schools for the training of health personnel. Such a procedure remains the exclusive prerogative of the national government concerned. The list of names in the WHO *World Directory of Medical Schools* is compiled from data received from or confirmed by member states. The organization does not accept responsibility for the inclusion or the omission of the names of any institutions.

If your school is not included in the directory at the time of your graduation, do not lose heart. Contact a member of your school administration to find out why the school is not included. Armed with this information, you can then approach the ECFMG, which promises to consider such instances on a case-by-case basis.

Another cautionary note deserves mention here. Entry into medical school is highly competitive around the globe. Attainment of the medical degree is viewed as an extremely desirable attribute by both students and their parents. These factors together have caused the number of medical schools to mushroom in some countries. Some of these medical schools may not be well recognized by various international agencies. So, while a degree earned at one of these medical schools may enable you to practice in your own country, it may not make you eligible for the USMLE.

MEDICAL EDUCATION CREDENTIALS

Effective July 1, 1998, an IMG must have at least four credit years in attendance at a medical school that is enrolled in the *World Directory of Medical Schools*. You are not required to have obtained an unrestricted license or certificate of registration to practice medicine in your country.

CREDENTIALING PROCESS

You are required to submit two copies of both sides of your medical school diploma along with two current full-face photographs to the ECFMG. If your medical diploma is not in English, you need to have it translated. This can be a problem in countries where recognized translating agencies are not easily locatable. Often, however, you can have the diploma translated by an official of your medical school. Do not forget to send the copies of the original along with the translation.

I have noticed that many IMGs do not send these credentialing documents along with their initial USMLE applications. This might be because these papers are not needed to enroll for the exam. However, such procrastination should be avoided, because getting the verification from your school can sometimes be a very lengthy process. ECFMG will normally let you know when they send the required papers to your medical school for verification. In some instances, you may have to approach your school officials to expedite the process.

APPLICATION PROCESS

You can request an application form for the USMLE from ECFMG in the following ways:

- By writing them at:
  ECFMG
  3624 Market St.
  Philadelphia, PA 19104 USA
- By fax: 215-387-9863.

- By visiting the public affairs office of any U.S. embassy or consulate around the world.
- By calling toll-free: 800-500-8249, from within the United States, or 215-375-1913 from anywhere in the world.

Calling the United States from other countries can be very expensive. When you dial the ECFMG's number, you may hear a computerized message that will guide you through a series of options. It may be difficult to understand and follow along with this message at first. As you try to understand the phone commands and punch or dial the numbers at the same time, you are no doubt thinking about the telephone charges that are accumulating as each minute passes. Here are a few time and money-saving tips:

- You may be connected immediately to a representative. If not, you will be connected to an automated message which begins: "Thank you for calling ECFMG. . . ." You do not have to listen to the whole of this message. Just punch or dial 1 (as per the menu at the time of writing this book) on your phone. That way, you will not have to spend time listening to a message that will tell you to punch or dial 1 anyway. This step will connect you to a representative who will take down your address.
- Usually, you will have to hold until a representative is available. To avoid this delay, call when it is Saturday or Sunday in the United States (these are not workdays in the United States). The waiting time is likely to be less on these days.
- When a representative comes on the phone, he or she knows you are calling to request an application. Just say "I am calling to request an application form for the USMLE," and when asked, proceed to give your address, spelling each word. This will help the operator, who may not be familiar with your accent, to understand you.

These simple steps should help save you money.

COMPLETING THE APPLICATION FORM

To register for the USMLE steps 1 or 2, you must send the completed application form along with a fee, to ECFMG. The form has four main parts (A–D) and is fairly straightforward. Five areas that are likely to confuse IMGs are explained below:

- **Part A, column 1.** ECFMG/USMLE number: When you apply to take the exam for the first time, you are allotted an identification number. This number helps ECFMG direct all of your correspondence to the same file, and it is retained even if you cancel your registration. You are supposed to enter this ID number at the top of the application form. It is very important that you use the original ID number that is allotted to you for all subsequent applications. Multiple ID numbers can give rise to a lot of confusion and can result in the loss of your application form, fee, or other correspondence.
- **Part B, column 10.3.** Clinical clerkships: Medical students in the United States perform hospital rotations called clinical clerkships. Medical students throughout the world also complete such hospital rotations during medical school. Simply fill in the time you spent in the different specialties. IMGs from those countries that require a mandatory internship be completed before awarding a medical degree can write the time spent in different specialties during their rotating internship.
- **Part B, column 11.** Medical licensure: Here you are supposed to give details of any license you have received to practice medicine in your country. According to new rules, you are no longer required to have an unrestricted license from your own country to be eligible to take the USMLE 1 or 2.
- **Part B, column 12.** Hospital training: While filling out this column, remember that the form is only used to evaluate your eligibility for the exams. I have seen some IMGs with long medical professional histories try to cram all of this information into this column. These details are not necessary. Just fill in the major residency or fellowship training you completed.
- **Part C, column 19.1; B.1.** Here you are asked to explain why the application form could not be signed in the presence of your medical school dean. Be truthful. If you are far away from your medical school and think that traveling there will be difficult, say so. Explain any other reasons for not being able to return to your medical school to have the form signed.

PAYING THE USMLE FEE

The fee that accompanies the USMLE application must be paid in U.S. dollars. IMGs from countries that have so-called open currencies do not have any problem with this. They can go to any bank in their country, obtain the required amount of dollars, and send them in the form of a check or money order to ECFMG. IMGs from countries that do not have open currencies have a problem, however, because they cannot buy dollars. If you are in this situation, one solution is to ask someone you know who lives in another country or in the United States to send the fee on your behalf. If you do this, be sure to tell the person sending the fee to write your USMLE ID number on the check, otherwise, ECFMG cannot credit the payment properly to your account.

STEP 1: THE EXAM

According to the information bulletin published by the USMLE, "Step 1 assesses whether you can apply the knowledge and understanding of key concepts of basic biomedical science, with an emphasis on the principles and mechanism of health, disease and mode of therapy." Most IMGs are more apprehensive about taking step 1 than step 2. This is usually because these IMGs have been away from medical school for several years before they apply to take step 1. Biochemistry, in particular, seems to scare a lot of IMGs. However, several good books are available that can make even a subject such as biochemistry interesting. Choose the books that suit your style of studying.

PASS/FAIL STATISTICS

The pass/fail statistics for IMGs are shown in Table 4–1.

TABLE 4–1. Number of International Medical Graduates Tested and Percent Passing the USMLE Step 1 in 1998

	June 1998		October 1998		1998 Total	
IMG Registrants	No. Tested	% Passing	No. Tested	% Passing	No. Tested	% Passing
First-time takers	8392	66	5204	56	13,596	62
Repeaters	6479	33	4167	30	10,646	32
Total IMGs	14,871	52	9371	45	24,242	49

Source: National Board of Medical Examiners, at *www.nbme.org*

COURSE OUTLINES

Following are the subjects you need to study for the USMLE 1:

- ❑ Biochemistry
- ❑ Anatomy
- ❑ Physiology
- ❑ Pharmacology
- ❑ Microbiology
- ❑ Pathology
- ❑ Behavioral sciences

For those of you interested in statistics, you are required to answer 55 to 65 percent of the questions correctly to pass. I personally do not believe in these numbers. My reasoning is that, being an IMG, in the competitive environment of the United States, you should not just be thinking of passing. You will need good scores to get into a good residency program. Therefore, for the purpose of taking the board exam, I recommend that you have good grasp of the required subject areas. I also recommend that you prepare by reading good board review books. These books tend to focus your attention on the topics that are most relevant from the standpoint of the exam. This is a great help for IMGs. One other thing you are expected to be knowledgeable about is application of the basic sciences.

TOPICS LIKELY TO BE OVERLOOKED BY IMGs

A thorough knowledge of all aspects of acquired immunodeficiency syndrome (AIDS) is very important. After you have thoroughly studied all of the subjects on the course outline, check to be sure you have a detailed understanding of the following topics.

Biochemistry

This subject scares almost all of the IMGs preparing for step 1. There are three main reasons for this phenomenon:

1. Most of the IMGs have been away from medical school for some time when they sit for the examination. They are typically

practicing in a field of medicine that does not involve direct use of the concepts taught in biochemistry.

2. All medical schools teach biochemistry at the start of training. This typically is the time when you get into medical school and want to celebrate your hard-earned entry. Some medical students are likely to be less serious about studies during the first couple of years of school.
3. The clinical importance of biochemistry cannot be appreciated until a physician starts to work in the clinical fields. Since this subject is taught to medical students early in their training, before they have seen a real patient, it may appear to be simply a bunch of dreary formulas. (This problem occurs with all of the basic subjects.)

Think of biochemistry concepts as they apply to clinical medicine. This can help make an otherwise dull and drab (for most of the people) subject interesting.

Let me illustrate by using the example of a very intelligent friend of mine who was accepted into an orthopedics residency. Shortly thereafter he began going to the dissection hall to perform the dissection of cadavers. He explained this to me by saying that if he had realized the importance of having a detailed understanding of basic human anatomy during his first year of medical school, he would have been more attentive in the dissection sessions then. I had a somewhat similar experience while rereading the basic subjects in preparation for the USMLE exam. Just revisiting these subjects helped to explain many things in the clinical practice of medicine that I had been puzzled about. An awareness of these basic aspects of various clinical problems helps one think at a higher level as compared to others. It also improves the versatility of one's thought process.

Once you begin to appreciate the clinical importance of these basic subjects, preparation for step 1 can become more enjoyable and effective. A flexible approach to studying may also help you avoid horror stories like the following which was told to me by a friend: "I married a girl and came to North America. After a few days of celebrating our arrival here, I decided to sit down to begin studying. I started with biochemistry. For the next 5 days, I could not get beyond page 1. There I was, sitting by myself in a room, while my wife of only a few days and her relatives thought I was studying. I tried sleeping, without success. On the fifth day, I cried. I just could not study. I could see no way out of this depression until one of my new friends told me that I should forget about biochemistry and start with pharmacology. It worked for me." Today, my friend is a successful physician employed by a well-respected university.

The following list outlines selected topics in biochemistry that are important in many clinical situations. This list is not meant to be comprehensive. Rather, it is provided with the sole aim of stimulating your interest in the subject.

- The Henderson-Hasselbalch equation, which will help you understand acid–base balance in the body.
- Basic concepts of enzyme activity, which are essential to everyday practice.
- The role of vitamins and the various biochemical reactions that specific vitamins take part in. This knowledge is indispensable for diagnosing and treating many disease states. Vitamin D metabolism is affected by several disease states of the kidney and liver, and vitamin K plays an important role in the coagulation system of your patients.
- Various cycles, such as the tricarboxylic acid cycle and glycolysis, which will help you understand the physiological and pathological states of your patients. You must know the various enzymes and co-factors involved at different steps of the cycles. You should also know the energy bonds generated or consumed at different steps.
- Diseases caused by various enzyme deficiencies, such as lactose deficiency, galactosemia, and glucose-6-phosphate dehydrogenase (G6PD) deficiency.
- Glycogen storage diseases, sphingolipidosis, and others.
- The structure of the heme and oxygen dissociation curve, which will help you in solving many of the complex problems affecting patients in the intensive care unit (ICU).
- The rate-limiting steps of various biochemical and metabolic cycles, such as cholesterol synthesis.
- The importance of cholesterol synthesis and lipid absorption. This cannot be overemphasized, as during your years in the United States, you will be dealing with a population that has a high incidence of coronary artery disease.
- Details of DNA and RNA activity, including replication, translation, synthesis, and so on. Genetics is the wave of the future. The etiologies of many diseases are coming down to genes. Genetic engineering is likely to provide a cure for many diseases in the future. Gene therapy is showing some promise in revascularization. A thorough knowledge of genetics is therefore likely to be a

necessary prerequisite for the coming generation (your generation) of doctors.

Now, choose a good biochemistry book and sit down to read it. Once you understand the importance of this subject, reading about biochemistry will never be drudgery again.

Anatomy

Most of the test questions will focus on topics in anatomy that are likely to be clinically important. Consider reading a concise review of neuroanatomy.

Physiology

Acid–Base Balance and Kidney Function.

- The anion gap and its importance
- Interpretation of arterial blood gases
- Tubular secretion and reabsorption
- Glomerular filtration and its mechanism

Blood. Awareness that neutrophils are called segments or segs, and immature segs are called bands. Thus, if a question reports high levels of bands, this indicates increased neutrophil maturation in the bone marrow with release of immature forms due to the increased activity (the so-called "left shift").

- Different type of blood reactions and their management
- Sickle cell anemia
- High-tech modalities used in the treatment of various hematological malignancies. Once again, in answering a question you should not pick the most technologically advanced modality unless you know it to be of proven benefit, as referenced in one of your books.

Cardiovascular System. The action potential curve of the myocyte and the changes at the cellular level at different stages.

- The cardiac cycle
- Autoregulation of blood
- Exercise physiology

- The mechanism of hypertension and various antihypertensive medications that act at different levels
- The physiology of heart failure and the mechanism of action of different therapeutic modalities

Respiratory System. Pulmonary volumes

- Pulmonary function tests
- The oxygen dissociation curve
- The 0_2 and CO_2 transport system
- Sleep apnea
- High-altitude physiology

Central Nervous System. Different nerve tracts and their pathways

- Motor, sensory and cerebellar systems
- Cranial nerves
- Bladder control

Gastrointestinal Tract. Hormones: their functions

- Control mechanisms of various gastric secretions
- The mechanism of ulcer formation, and the role of *Helicobacter pylori*
- Different stages of digestion and various pathological states
- Vitamins

Endocrinology. Major hormones: their functions and diseases resulting from hypo- or hypersecretion

- Sex hormones and ways to diagnose different pathological states
- Male impotence and infertility
- Female infertility
- Physiology of pregnancy

Pharmacology

- Medication side effects that are most likely to be seen in everyday practice
- The drug of choice for different clinical situations, and various factors that affect the choice

- The questions do not usually test knowledge of medication doses unless the dosage prescribed is an issue on its own; for example, dopamine has different effects at different doses.
- Issues relating to polypharmacy. In the United States, with the advent of subspecialization, many patients—especially elderly—end up receiving prescriptions for medications from several physicians. Some questions may require you to analyze whether a patient needs to be taken off particular drugs rather than prescribed additional medications.
- Drugs for the geriatric population
- The analgesics of choice in different clinical situations, and their side effects
- First-line medications for different types of hypertensive patients; for example, an African-American patient, a patient with coronary artery disease, a patient with diabetes mellitus, and so forth
- Antiarrhythmics and their common side effects
- Myocardial infarction: Pharmacotherapy, and knowledge of "what to do, when"
- Asthma: Awareness of the algorithmic approach
- Treatment of peptic ulcer along with that of *H. pylori*
- The most common antineoplastic agents and their side effects
- The drug of choice for various infections, and the second choice in case the patient is allergic to the first-line drug
- Various groups of antibiotics
- Anticonvulsants
- Signs and symptoms of drug abuse and specific types of drug overdoses
- Symptoms and long-term effects of various illicit drugs and their management; for example, coronary disease secondary to cocaine use
- Drug rehabilitation programs

Microbiology

- The clinical spectrum of diseases caused by different organisms and ways to diagnose and treat them
- The prevalence of different organisms according to geographical distribution within the United States or around the world (*Hint:* sometimes a clue is provided by the stated location in the question)
- Immunology
- Major fungal, spirochetal, bacterial, and viral diseases

Pathology

I have no specific recommendation here, but I would suggest you review an atlas of pathology slides, in addition to reading a review book.

Behavioral Sciences

Webster's dictionary describes behavioral science as a science—such as psychology—that deals with human action and seeks to generalize about human behavior in society. Most IMGs do not learn this as a specific subject in the medical school. Although this is a somewhat commonsense subject, you should understand the basic concepts behind the behavioral sciences. This will probably require only light reading for majority of IMGs. Topics that should receive extra attention are the following:

- Interpersonal relationships
- Ego defense mechanisms
- The grief reaction
- The physician–patient relationship
- Stages of sleep and drugs that depress rapid eye movement (REM) sleep, such as barbiturates, alcohol, phenothiazines, and monoamine oxidase (MAO) inhibitors. (*Note:* the benzodiazepines do not cause rebound of REM sleep)

WHAT IF I FAIL?

If one fails the examination, one's first step before hitting the books again should be to review exam preparation strategy to identify areas that need to be improved.

Candidates who fail the USMLE 1 should take some time off before beginning the process of studying to retake the exam. First take a long, critical look at your style of studying. Next, ask yourself whether you really understand the "soul of the exam" (see Chapter 3). Are you reading the right kinds of books? Make sure you are not wasting too much time by trying to read bulky textbooks. On the other hand, you might be relying on books that deal with the exam topics at a too-superficial level.

The percentages of examinees who passed the USMLE 1 on another attempt after a failure are shown in Table 4–2. I have included this table to drive home the point that the chances of passing on the second attempt decrease in direct proportion to the score on the failed exam.

If you fail the exam, your first reaction may be to go back and bury your head in your books. For many IMGs who fail, this may be the first major failure of their lives, which can give rise to a lot of anger and anguish. My research shows that for many of these IMGs, returning to the books with a greater vehemence is their main form of psychological release. While this may be the right strategy in some other situations, it may not be the best thing to do in this particular situation. Keep in mind that this is not a type of exam that you have had experience with to this point in your life. It is an exam given to you by a foreign system of testing, and you are trying to prove yourself adequate according to standards set by a foreign agency. Remember that you have failed in subjects that you had already passed during your medical school training. Thus, there is a high probability that your preparation strategy might be at fault, not your knowledge base. Try to understand the soul of this exam on the basis of the information provided in this book. I think the cause of failure for a significant number of IMGs is not a lack of knowledge, but rather a lack of awareness of how to apply that knowledge to the American-style practice of medicine.

TABLE 4–2. Performance of Step 1 Repeaters: October 1998 Pass Rate of NBME-registered Repeaters Who Failed Step 1 for the First Time in June 1998

June Scores	% Passing in October
176–178	85
173–175	76
170–172	66
165–169	52
160–164	33
150–159	12
<150	0
Total	60

Source: National Board of Medical Examiners, *www.nbme.org*.
Minimum passing score = 179.

CHAPTER 5

USMLE Step 2

ELIGIBILITY CRITERIA FOR STEP 2

To be eligible to take the USMLE step 2, you should be within 12 months of completing the full didactic curriculum. This means that you should not be more than 12 months away from graduating from medical school. But this begs the question, why would you want to sit for the USMLE 2 in the final year of medical school when you have not even finished studying the subjects that you are likely to be tested on? IMGs who have to complete a compulsory rotatory internship before they graduate are in a better position, as they can take step 2 while they are still interns. Your medical school should be included in the WHO *World Directory of Medical Schools*, as explained in Chapter 4.

APPLICATION PROCESS

The method for requesting an application and registering for the exam is the same as for step 1. The same form is used for both steps.

STEP 2: THE EXAM

Step 2 is designed to assess your ability to apply the medical knowledge that you have acquired in medical school. The knowledge tested is that considered essential for providing the patient care under supervision. A significant emphasis is given to health promotion and preventive medicine. Overall, this test requires you to demonstrate the ability to practice medicine safely.

Most IMGs feel more confident about taking step 2 than step 1 for the reasons enumerated in Chapter 4. Many excellent books designed to help prepare for the USMLE 2 are available. Choose those that best suit your style of studying.

More than step 1, this is a test that IMGs are likely to fail for a lack of understanding of the soul of the exam. You will have to tailor your study style to the demands of the exam before you can expect to do well. I am stressing this point for two reasons:

Evaluate how your style of practicing medicine compares to that prevalent in the United States.

1. The practice of medicine in the United States differs in many ways from that in other countries around the world. IMGs from other countries must understand these differences if they are to do well on this test, which evaluates application of their medical knowledge.
2. Many IMGs, before coming to the United States, have already begun practicing medicine in their own countries. This may be in the form of a residency or some type of private practice. The time spent in their country tends to mold their style of practice over time. This style, while useful and appropriate to the practice of medicine in their own country, may not hold them in good stead when they have to sit for a test designed to meet American standards.

PASS/FAIL STATISTICS

The pass/fail statistics for IMGs are shown in Table 5–1.

COURSE OUTLINES

Following are the subjects you need to study for the USMLE 2:

- ❏ Obstetrics and gynecology
- ❏ Psychiatry
- ❏ Pediatrics
- ❏ Preventive medicine and public health
- ❏ Internal medicine
- ❏ Surgery

COMPENSATING FOR DIFFERENT TEACHING STYLES

For step 2, not only will you need to study some good board review books, but you will also have to cultivate a certain style of practicing

TABLE 5-1. Number of International Medical Graduates Tested and Percent Passing the USMLE 2 in 1997–1998

	August 1997		March 1998		1997–1998 Total	
IMG Registrants	**No. Tested**	**% Passing**	**No. Tested**	**% Passing**	**No. Tested**	**% Passing**
First-time takers	8013	58	12,943	54	20,956	55
Repeaters	6199	41	7936	32	14,135	36
Total IMGs	14,212	50	20,879	46	35,091	48

Source: National Board of Medical Examiners, at *www.nbme.org*.

medicine. I recommend that you take your cues from the chapters in this book and begin to cultivate this style in readiness for taking step 2, step 3, and the CSA.

On the following pages, I enumerate the important subjects to be covered. Before I begin, I want to make a point. After having been trained in the British style and working in the American system for several years, I have noted some differences in the teaching styles of these two systems. For example, during my British style years, if my professor asked me to read up on mitral stenosis (MS), I would know that he expected me to memorize 15 causes of MS and to know 10 echocardiographic features, with some knowledge of different aspects of management. If I were asked to prepare the same topic in the United States, however, I would again be expected to know the common causes and clinical features of MS, but I would also be expected to know about the plan for antibiotic prophylaxis, follow up of the patient, and referral to a cardiologist.

As this simple example reveals, in the British style of teaching, you are expected to have both a good recall of clinical facts and an awareness of uncommon conditions, called "zebras" in American slang. On the positive side, you end up knowing a lot about every topic. On the negative side, even though you know a lot about a topic, you may not be able to apply all of that knowledge in a real-life situation.

In contrast, in the American style of teaching, you are expected to know how to diagnose and treat common conditions. I think of the United States as the land of algorithms. Doctors trained in the United States, while they may not be equipped to impress others with their knowledge of rare syndromes, are well equipped to avoid committing dangerous acts of omission or commission in everyday practice. The philosophy behind this approach is that you should be able to diagnose common problems, and if you are caught among zebras once in a while, you can always go back to your books. In the United States, it is common to see professors referring to a book in front of their residents or students. In contrast, I remember one incident involving one of my friends who was a senior resident in Pakistan at the time. He was "caught" referring to his book while treating a patient with diabetic ketoacidosis. As a result, he lost the respect of all of his junior residents overnight. A senior resident having to refer to a book to treat a patient? Ultimate sacrilege!

TOPICS LIKELY TO BE OVERLOOKED BY IMGs

The following list is provided with the understanding that you will be studying a good book on each of the subjects enumerated in the course outline.

Obstetrics and Gynecology

- *Female hormones:* Their importance in pregnant and nonpregnant patients and in some pathological states.
- *Pregnancy and the puerperium:* Knowledge of these aspects that will enable you to manage a normal pregnancy and delivery. You should also be knowledgeable about the normal pueperium and pathological states during this period.
- *Antepartum care:* The United States has a high incidence of teenage pregnancies, and there are often compliance and social issues with these young patients. These issues could be a new experience for IMGs from certain countries.
- *Fetal well-being:* In the United States, there is a trend toward aggressive fetal monitoring. As a prospective internist, you may not know the finer details of these modalities, but you should be knowledgeable about conditions where such monitoring is warranted.
- *Pregnant patients with other medical conditions:* You should know the exact plan for pregnant patients with diabetes, hypertension, urinary tract infection (UTI), and so on. Think about such a patient coming to your clinic, and imagine the knowledge that you would need to have to be able to take care of this patient safely.

- *Identification of high-risk patients:* Knowledge of the criteria for referral to a specialist.
- *Antepartum complications:* The ability to readily diagnose and manage various complications.
- *Teratology:* Knowledge of the teratogenic effects of various environmental agents on the fetus, and an understanding of how to modify the treatment of choice for various disease states in view of such effects.
- *Adolescent gynecology:* In view of the high incidence of teenage sexual activity, you should be able to diagnose and adequately treat sexually transmitted diseases.
- *Family planning:* This includes counseling for young females.
- *Pelvic pain:* You are expected to be aware of life-threatening conditions such as ectopic pregnancy.
- *Abortion:* This is a very sensitive issue in the United States. I would suggest almost never should you choose elective abortion as the correct answer on the exam.
- *Menopause:* Knowledge of well-recognized strategies for hormone replacement.
- *Malignancies:* Knowledge of the algorithmic approach to the management of different malignancies.
- *Vaginitis* and the differential diagnosis of various etiologies on the basis of discharge characteristics and smear examination.
- *Dysfunctional uterine bleeding* and postmenopausal bleeding.
- *Hirsutism.*
- *Health promotion and preventive medicine* as applied to gynecology and obstetrics.

Psychiatry

This is another Achilles' heel for many IMGs. The reasons for this are several:

Along with physical health, pay attention to the mental (psychiatric and psychological) health of your patients. This will help you do better with test items related to psychiatry.

- Students in most countries around the world spend only a few weeks learning about psychiatry during medical school.
- Psychiatric questions constitute a very small percentage of test questions during their medical school years.
- Subtle psychiatric problems are neither well comprehended nor well managed in most countries with limited resources. Since

the practice of medicine in such countries does not necessitate knowledge of psychiatry, most IMGs do not have much experience with this field.

As you are studying in preparation for taking the board exam, it will help to imagine the specific conditions in the form of patients at your clinic. Most of the test questions on psychiatry will be in form of vignettes. Remember that the focus of the questions is on issues related to everyday practice, not the theoretical knowledge quickly acquired from the pages of a review book. While focusing your study in this way, you may also recall patients from your past experience who now begin to fit into these diagnoses. Continue this approach as you review other subjects for the exam.

Be sure you are knowledgeable about the following topics:

- *History and clinical examination of a psychiatric patient:* I think this is the most important aspect. Once you understand the way to interview a psychiatric patient and to perform the mental status examination, half the battle is won. This knowledge will help you understand important features of different clinical conditions.
- *Psychiatric therapies:* It is important to know the basic features of the common therapies used in psychiatric care, and the different conditions for which they may be beneficial.
- *Subtlety:* You should be able to appreciate subtle features of major psychiatric disorders and common features of subtle psychiatric disorders. Remember, the main purpose for these questions is to test your ability to diagnose and manage such patients in your practice. This aspect is usually somewhat difficult for IMGs because internists in our countries are generally not trained to catch subtle hints of mental illness. Additionally, some psychiatric problems are unique to the United States and may not be prevalent in the countries where most IMGs were trained.
- *Personality disorders:* Think about people you know who may fit the different personality types. This may help you understand these concepts.
- *Psychiatric emergencies:* You should be able to recognize various emergencies and be able to act as warranted.
- *Common topics:*
  - Delirium and dementia
  - Major depression
  - Cyclothymia
  - Bipolar disorder
  - Hypomania
  - Somatoform and panic disorders
  - Schizophrenia
  - Indications for electroconvulsive therapy (ECT)
  - Posttraumatic stress disorder

Pediatrics

Most of the IMGs I interviewed in preparing this book stated that they "just read something on neonatology" when studying for the exam, and they did not think they missed much by not formally preparing for this subject. If you do not have a lot of time at hand, I think it is okay to just read up on neonatology. Most of the books on internal medicine also tend to cover diseases of slightly older children, partly because most of these diseases tend to carry over into the young adolescent population.

Preventive Medicine and Public Health

This is an interesting and important subject, the main concept of which is the same as that of its counterpart in other countries. The difference is that this time you will be reading about the realities of the United States. Even if this was not a subject that IMGs are tested on, I would still recommend every IMG read a book on this subject. By doing so, you will learn about the main health problems in the United States and the efforts to deal with them. Most books on this subject will also include statistics on medical practice patterns in the United States. After taking this exam, you may not be able to pinpoint the questions that seemed to belong to the area of social and preventive medicine; most of these questions are well woven into other subjects. The following are some of the topics you should be familiar with:

- *Leading causes of death* in different age groups in the United States.
- *Reportable diseases* in the United States: these are AIDS, tuberculosis, syphilis, salmonella, shigella, gonorrhea, chicken pox, mumps, measles, rubella, and hepatitis A and B.
- *Screening:* You should know about various screening tests recommended, the age groups that should receive them, and the frequency of such tests.
- *Substance abuse.*
- *Family planning.*
- The *relative importance of different health problems* in the United States.

Internal Medicine

- *Preoperative evaluation.*
- *Geriatrics:* In the United States, the elderly make up a very high percentage of the population. Some older adults live on their

The geriatric population has its own unique problems, which demand an approach specially tailored for this group.

own in the community. Others are supported by their families to varying degrees. Yet others are in long-term care facilities. With age, some of the mental faculties decline. It is important to be aware of these realities. If you understand this, it is easy to understand the problems of this population. Special points to ponder are as follows:

- Abuse of older people
- Polypharmacy
- Examination of the older population, including mental evaluation
- Immobility and instability
- Patients' ability to take medications regularly and in the right dose

- *Hematology:*
  - Sickle cell anemia is an important disease, especially in the African-American population
  - Awareness of different causes of anemia in various patient populations in the United States; the diagnostic algorithm and way to manage different types of anemia
  - Coagulation disorders

- *Neurology:*
  - Dementia
  - Latest standard of management of stroke
  - Diagnosis of migraine
  - Presentation of subdural hematoma in the older population

- *Cardiology:*
  - Management of dyslipidemia
  - Thorough knowledge of various aspects of coronary artery disease and congestive heart failure
  - Physical findings in various valvular diseases
  - Management of common tachy- and bradyarrhythmias

- *Respiratory Diseases:*
  - Management of chronic obstructive pulmonary disease (COPD)
  - The algorithmic approach to the management of asthma
  - Respiratory failure and its management
  - Epiglottitis

- Lung cancer: Different types, staging, and management
- In-depth knowledge of various management aspects of deep venous thrombosis and pulmonary embolism

- *Nephrology:*
  - The relative prevalence of various renal diseases in different patient populations
  - Renal failure and dialysis: The United States has a large population receiving chronic dialysis. These patients are usually followed by internists for everyday problems. The knowledge of various aspects of care of a patient with renal failure on chronic dialysis is required.
  - Electrolytes: Calculation of water deficit on the basis of sodium level and other deficits on the basis of serum level (e.g., bicarbonate)

- *Endocrinology:*
  - Detailed knowledge of management aspects of diabetes mellitus
  - Various causes of hyponatremia
  - Syndrome of inappropriate antidiuretic hormone (SIADH)
  - Pituitary and hypothalamic disorders
  - Interpretation of thyroid function tests; diagnosis of various thyroid diseases

- *Infectious diseases:*
  - Human immunodeficiency virus (HIV) infection.

- *Rheumatology:*
  - Knowledge of the diagnostic value of joint fluid aspirate
  - Systemic associates of various rheumatological disorders
  - Tests for different conditions based on their sensitivity and specificity

- *Dermatology:*
  - The ability to diagnose common dermatological problems by seeing a photograph or on the basis of a description
  - Skin diseases associated with various systemic diseases

- *Gastroenterology:*
  - Alcoholic liver disease
  - Inflammatory bowel diseases

Surgery

- *Trauma:* Awareness of the algorithmic approach to a patient with trauma.
- *Fluid management.*
- *Care of postoperative complications.*
- *Surgery in patients with other medical conditions.*
- *Basic knowledge of anesthesia.*
- *Malignancies:* The ability to stage different malignancies on the basis of information given in a vignette, and awareness of management strategy according to the stage.
- *Management of acute abdomen and life-threatening hemorrhage.*
- *Orthopedics:* Awareness of common problems and their management.
- *ENT and ophthalmology:* Knowledge of simple concepts.

WHAT IF I FAIL?

The percentage of examinees who pass the USMLE 2 on another attempt after a failure are shown in Table 5–2. In the unfortunate event of a failure on this exam, one should reevaluate one's preparation strategy, as described in Chapter 4.

TABLE 5–2. Performance of Step 2 Repeaters: March 1998 Pass Rate of NBME-registered Repeaters Who Failed Step 2 for the First Time in August 1997

August Score	% Passing in March
167–169	91
164–166	93
159–163	80
150–158	57
<150	25
Total	72

Source: National Board of Medical Examiners, *www.nbme.org.*
Minimum passing score = 170.

CHAPTER 6

English Exam (TOEFL)

The reasonable ability to understand spoken English as well as the ability to communicate in this language are essential prerequisites prior to assuming patient care responsibility in a graduate medical education program in the United States. The English exam is designed to test this ability in IMGs.

This test is usually quite easy for IMGs from countries where English is taught from an early age. Apart from getting used to the American pronunciation and accent, these IMGs do not have to put much extra effort into passing the exam. However, IMGs from countries where English is not taught can have substantial difficulties with this test.

THE IMPORTANCE OF HAVING A GOOD GRASP OF ENGLISH

The ability to speak and understand English is an important but sometimes overlooked factor influencing your career in the United States.

You should critically evaluate your ability to both understand and speak English. By this I do not mean that you need to acquire the type of accent appropriate for an anchorperson on CNN. Rather, you need to evaluate whether you will be able to get your point across while conversing with an average American. I have found that the English test seems to be the last of the priorities of most IMGs trying to come to the United States. IMGs who feel they are weak in English do tend to work harder, but their efforts seem to be accurately titrated to enable them to just barely pass this test. If you think you have a problem understanding or speaking English, start working hard to improve your ability now. Do not venture into the medical field in the United States until you are confident that you can communicate reasonably well in English. You must do this, even if it means working an extra year on your English. Sounds crazy? Read on.

Hundreds of IMGs who are working full time in United States research labs would much prefer to be practicing clinical medicine. Research is a highly respected field; however, you should not be forced into a position of having to do this work if you do not want to. Among those who are forced to work in research labs are some IMGs who could not pass their USMLE tests. Another subgroup is there because they can neither understand nor write nor speak English well. Many of these individuals have the medical credentials to be able to enter a residency program in the United States. This is a tragic situation, especially when you consider that these people—who have learned everything from the structure of humeral bone to blood gas analysis—are held back because of their inability to learn a language. It should not have to happen.

As of March 3, 1999, TOEFL is the only formal test of English language proficiency for IMGs.

TYPES OF TESTS

As of March 3, 1999, the ECFMG English test (EET) is no longer being offered; the test for English proficiency is now the TOEFL (Test of English as a Foreign Language), and it is a necessary step toward ECFMG certification. The main differences between TOEFL and the old EET are as follows:

1. TOEFL began to be computerized, starting in July 1998, and there is a plan to phase in computerization of this test completely by 2001. The test is now given on computers at several locations. At the time of writing this book, however, the Educational Testing Service (ETS) has had logistical problems implementing the computerized test in some places in the world. As a result, some locations may continue to offer the pencil-and-paper exam until the computerization process is complete. Check the latest information from ETS before taking the test. The pros and one con of the computerized test are summarized in Table 6–1.
2. One section of the exam that did not have a counterpart in the EET is the test of written English (TWE). This involves writing a short essay on a given subject (see later discussion).

If you are taking TOEFL for the purpose of ECFMG certification or recertification, you must also do the following:

TABLE 6–1. Pros and Con of the Computerized TOEFL

Pros

- You will have the ability to control the speed of the audio feed, as you deem fit. But beware, you still have a limited amount of time to complete the test.
- The reporting of the test results will be faster.

Con

- The computer-naïve test-taker: The administering organizations have done some research to see if computer naïveté is likely to affect test scores, and their research has reportedly shown no significant difference. However, even if the test-takers in the research sample were from different countries, they were more likely to be from the elite universities in the more famous cities of the world. (This is because these more famous institutions in bigger cities are more easily accessible to the researchers.) IMGs from such schools are likely to be more computer savvy than those from a smaller city.

- On the day of the TOEFL exam, request that the ETS submit your score to ECFMG. This can be done by entering the ECFMG institution code number—**9108**—on the mailing instruction form provided by the ETS. ECFMG will only accept the score if it comes directly from TOEFL. You must request that ETS report your TOEFL score directly to ECFMG.
- Pay the ECFMG a fee in dollars to accept your TOEFL score. Along with this payment, you should also send information specifying the date on which you took the exam, your full name (as it appears on both your ECFMG file and your TOEFL application), your USMLE number, and your ETS number. This will help ECFMG connect all of your paperwork.

You must request that ETS report your TOEFL score directly to ECFMG.

APPLICATION PROCESS

An application for this test can be requested in the following different ways:

- By writing to ETS at:
  Educational Testing Service
  Princeton, NJ 08541 USA
- By calling 609-771-7100.
- By e-mail at *toefl@ets.org*.

- On the Internet at *http://www.toefl.org*. You can download information along with the application form from this Web site. This form may not be useful in some countries. Look for the list of such countries on the Web site.
- By contacting a local center in some countries. Check to see if one is available in your country.

FEES

The computer-based TOEFL test fee is U.S.$100. The payment can be made by different methods and in different currencies. Check the information bulletin from ETS.

SCHEDULING

There are several different choices for scheduling, as described below.

FOR SCHEDULING IN THE UNITED STATES, CANADA, AMERICAN SAMOA, GUAM, THE UNITED STATES VIRGIN ISLANDS, AND PUERTO RICO

By Phone

You can call 800-468-6335 (only from within the United States) or 410-843-4862. You may also call from outside the previously mentioned areas to schedule the test at a center within the United States. You will be asked for the same information that is requested in the CBT voucher request form available in the information bulletin. Having all of this information handy will save time. You will be given all of the information that you need over the telephone. The ETS stresses that you should not mail or fax a scheduling form after telephone scheduling. This will result in your being scheduled and billed twice. The payment can be made by certain types of credit cards acceptable to ETS or by CBT voucher number.

How to Get a CBT Voucher You should fill in the form provided in the bulletin, make your payment by one of the methods accepted by the ETS, and mail both of these items to the ETS. According to the service, it should take 2 to 4 weeks for your voucher to be processed and mailed to you. (Of course, the time it takes for the mail to reach you may differ depending on where you live.) If you have already applied for a CBT voucher, you should not call to schedule the test before you receive the voucher. This can lead to double scheduling and double charging. The voucher is valid for 1 year. If you do not receive the voucher or you loose it after receiving it, call 609-771-7700 for help.

Walk-in Scheduling

You can walk into a center for same-day testing without a prior appointment. An appointment will depend on the availability. You should be ready to make your payment in one of the ways acceptable to the ETS and also to present a valid passport as identification.

FOR SCHEDULING OUTSIDE PREVIOUSLY MENTIONED AREAS

By Phone

You can call the appropriate regional registration center (RRC), as listed in the information bulletin. You will be asked all the information requested in the international test scheduling form. You should also be able to make payment by one of the methods acceptable to the ETS. This call must be made at least 3 business days prior to your preferred test date. You will be given all the information that you require over the telephone.

What Is an RRC? These centers have been established all across the world. Each RRC covers a group of test centers. The locations of various RRCs should be available in the information bulletin. You can also visit the official TOEFL Web site at *www.toefl.org* for the current list of centers. The bulletin states that if a center is not located within 200 kilometers of where you live and you cannot travel to take the test, you should contact the ETS to ask if special arrangements for testing can be made.

By Fax

You can fax the completed international test scheduling form, which should include the following information:

- Five date choices by month and day.
- The test center number of the center where you plan to take the test, and the name of the city where the center is located.
- Credit card information for payment. At the time of writing this book, the ETS accepted VISA®, MasterCard®, or the American Express® card.

You should fax the form to the appropriate RRC, as listed in the bulletin. The material must be received at least 7 days prior to your preferred test date. You will receive an appointment confirmation by fax or mail. If you do not receive your *preferred* date and the *assigned* date does not suit you, call the RRC within 24 hours of receipt of the confirmation information. If you do not receive the confirmation, you need to call RRC at least 3 business days prior to your first choice of test date to confirm your appointment status. According to the information in bulletin, the responsibility of finding this out rests with you.

By Mail

You need to send the same items as enumerated above; the only difference is that they should be mailed to the appropriate RRC. This material must be received at least 3 weeks before the first day of the earliest month you selected.

RESCHEDULING OR CANCELLATION OF AN APPOINTMENT

For candidates in the United States, Canada, American Samoa, Guam, the United States Virgin Islands, and Puerto Rico, the following steps are necessary:

1. You must call the center at 800-468-6335 no later than 3 days before your appointment. If you cancel, you will be given a partial refund. To reschedule, you will be charged a rescheduling fee of U.S.$20.
2. You will need to provide the appointment confirmation number and the full name that you used when you made the appointment.

Candidates in areas other than those listed above should follow a similar procedure except they should call the appropriate RRC instead.

POSITIVE IDENTIFICATION DOCUMENT

On the day of the exam, you will be asked to provide an acceptable form of identification. The ETS is very strict about this. You must have the type of identification document specified by ETS. The service has zero tolerance for those who diverge from the established policy in this regard.

You must have the type of identification document specified by ETS. The service has zero tolerance for those who diverge from the established policy in this regard.

- If you are visiting another country, you should have a passport; this serves as an acceptable ID document.
- In the absence of a passport, you should have one of the other documents that are acceptable to the ETS. Refer to the ETS information bulletin for a list of acceptable documents according to different countries.

If you have any doubt about the appropriateness of your ID document, call the RRC in advance to be sure it will be accepted.

HOW OFTEN CAN YOU TAKE THE TEST?

You can only take the computer-based test once a month, even if you cancelled the score of any test taken within this period. The TOEFL bulletin states that even if you manage to take the test twice within a month, your new score will not be released and you could be subjected to additional action. You cannot and should not try to take TOEFL more than once in a month.

You cannot and should not try to take TOEFL more than once in a month.

CANDIDATES WITH DISABILITIES

TOEFL offers wide range of accommodations for candidates with disabilities as long as the required documentation is provided by the applicant.

TOEFL: THE TEST

This is a multiple-choice examination. The computer-based TOEFL consists of four sections: (1) listening comprehension, (2) structure, (3) reading, and (4) test of written English.

LISTENING COMPREHENSION

In this section, you will listen to an audiotape recording of statements or conversation in everyday conversational English. At the end of each segment, you will be required to read the question printed in the test booklet and select the best response from a series of alternatives. In the computerized test, you will hear the conversation through headphones. This section tests your ability to understand simple English spoken with a common American accent. The importance of this part of the test cannot be overemphasized. Just consider that the only vehicle of communication between you and almost all of your patients in the United States is English. If you are not able to understand this type of conversation, how will you be able to interact with your patients?

The major feature of this section of the test is that it uses simple English. You do not have to pore over *Webster's* dictionary to be able to do well on this portion. Also, the testers do not expect you to understand someone speaking at the rate of a mile a minute. The speakers usually speak clearly and at a moderate pace.

STRUCTURE

This section is designed to gauge your ability to recognize language that is appropriate for standard written English. Following is a sample question appearing in this section of the TOEFL Bulletin:

> The Columbine flower, _______ to nearly all of the United States, can be raised from seed in almost any garden.
>
> - ❑ native
> - ❑ how native is
> - ❑ how native is it
> - ❑ is native

You have to decide which of the four choices should be chosen to fill in the blank to form a sensible sentence. The answer is "native."

READING

This section is designed to measure your understanding of standard written English. To do this, a written passage is provided and you are asked to answer questions based on the information given in the passage.

TWE: TEST OF WRITTEN ENGLISH

The TWE is a new feature of TOEFL.

In this section, you will be given a topic and asked to write a short essay on it. In the computer-based test, you have the option of typing or writing your essay. *Hint:* This is not a test of your philosophical position, so do not try to give the most politically correct opinion. The essay tests only your ability to communicate in writing. Refer to the information booklet for practice topics for this section.

PREPARING FOR TOEFL

Some IMGs have told me that they did not do anything in preparation for this exam. While I agree that it is possible to pass this test without any formal preparation, at the very least I would recommend you prepare by watching American videotapes. This could be in form of TV programs, movies, or educational videos (if available) from your school library. Listening to these tapes will help familiarize you with the American accent. This is one area where people who are already in the United States at the time they take the test are at an advantage. But do not get too worked up about the possibility that you won't understand the audio portion of the test. With a little practice, you will be fine.

If you are taking the computer-based test, you *must* become acquainted with the computer format of the test. You can gain experience using the sample provided by TOEFL. You can obtain this by the following methods:

You do not *have* to buy a CD-ROM but you should at least go through the sampler available on the Web, which is free of cost.

- Buying a CD-ROM.
- Downloading the tutorial and paying some money to the ETS.
- Watching it on the computer free of cost.

The tutorial has material on how to use a mouse, how to scroll, and examples of test items. I think anyone who spends any time on a computer should easily learn how to scroll and use the mouse; however, seeing examples of the test items on computer before you take the test can be very helpful.

If you think the TOEFL is likely to be difficult for you, consider signing up for a short-duration English course. One approach is to contact a major university in your area to ask if they offer courses in spoken English and listening comprehension of the language. I have done some research on the availability of these courses in different countries; the results are summarized in Table 6–2. If you are already in the

TABLE 6–2. Availability of English-Language Classes Worldwide

- English-language classes are available in quite a few countries, primarily in major cities. They are not always easily accessible, however, owing to geographical location.
- In some cases, the courses available may not suit the needs of an IMG who is planning to be a resident doctor in the United States.
- One positive trend that was uniformly noticed is that as many countries have begun to open their economic markets to the outside world, there has been a corresponding increase in the use of English. This should make English-language classes more readily available in these countries.
- The language departments of many universities are able to offer new classes in different languages if enough people are interested in joining the classes.

United States, contact a college or university in your area; most of them should offer English-language classes. Some high-schools or continuing education programs also offer English-as-a-second-language (ESL) classes.

My interviews with IMGs who failed the English test at least once provided the following stories:

- One of my friends from South America joined an English-language course in her area after coming to the United States. I had met her before she began the course. After a few weeks in the class, her ability to speak English had markedly improved. She not only passed the EET, but also turned out to be one of the most outgoing residents in her program. These achievements might not have been possible had she retained only a limited ability to speak English.
- Another friend, from India, told me he began paying more attention to the American accent after failing the test. He passed the next time.
- An IMG who clearly has a good command on English told another horror story. She dropped something from her desk in the middle of the listening comprehension section of the test. She missed one snippet of the audiotape and became so panicky that she was never able to synchronize the subsequent questions with the items in the answer book. The moral of this story—make sure you are ready before the start of listening comprehension part. And if you do miss something, forget about it and

move on. (Those of you who will take the test on computer will have control over the audio play, but you still need to avoid spending too much time on a single item.)

DURING THE EXAM

In the standard pencil-and-paper exam, once the audiotape for the listening comprehension portion of the test begins to play, it will not be interrupted. Apart from the ability to comprehend, this also is a test of concentration. After hearing each item, you have a few seconds to read the question and mark the answer. At the end of allotted time, the next item will begin to play regardless of whether or not you have finished the previous item. For these reasons, before this section of the test begins, check for any annoying or distracting sounds around you. If present, report these to the proctor before the tape starts. (These problems are likely to be eliminated with the computerized exam.)

REPEATING THE ENGLISH PROFICIENCY TEST

If you cannot gain admittance to a residency program within 2 years of passing the English exam, you must retake it.

THE NEXT STEP

Once you have passed the TOEFL along with the USMLE 1 and 2, you are eligible to take the clinical skills assessment (CSA) examination. Information about this exam is provided in Chapter 7.

CHAPTER 7

Clinical Skills Assessment Exam

After you have passed the USMLE steps 1 and 2 and the English proficiency test (TOEFL), the Clinical Skills Assessment (CSA) is the last examination that you must pass before receiving ECFMG certification. The CSA is a 1-day test currently administered in only one location: Philadelphia, Pennsylvania, in the United States. This test was added as one of the prerequisites of ECFMG certification in July 1998.

STATED PURPOSE OF THE CSA

According to ECFMG, "The purpose of CSA is to ensure that graduates of foreign medical schools can demonstrate the ability to gather and interpret clinical patient data, and communicate effectively on the English level comparable to students graduating from U.S. medical schools accredited by the Liaison Committee on Medical Education (LCME)."

For years, ECFMG worked to develop a CSA prototype that would provide an objective and consistent evaluation of the readiness of IMGs to enter graduate medical education programs in the United States. Various studies were conducted to assess the feasibility of conducting a reliable and valid test of clinical competence. ECFMG believes that the current test serves this purpose. The need for such a test stemmed from the different standards of training represented by IMGs from over 1400 medical schools worldwide who annually applied to enter U.S. residency programs. Before the CSA, there was no test for clinical competence or ability to communicate in English.

Testing using standardized patients, which is a feature of the CSA, has also been suggested as an examination method for students in U.S. medical schools. According to ECFMG, an objective, structured clinical examination is now in use in 60 percent of U.S. medical schools.

ISSUES SURROUNDING THE CSA

IMG PERSPECTIVE ON THE TEST

As noted, the CSA is a recent addition to the steps required to obtain ECFMG certification. This has been met with mixed feelings by many IMGs. I interviewed several IMGs about their views on the introduction of this test. The people I interviewed were at different levels of training in the United States. The prevalent feeling is summarized in the following paragraph: "The CSA has been devised as a step toward halting the entry of IMGs into the United States. The USMLE steps 1 and 2 are objective tests because computers know only one right answer to each question. So you are either right or wrong. There is no room for bias. But with the CSA, you have IMGs coming from other countries with a limited command of English. They are expected to perform a history and physical examination while talking with the typical (standardized) American patient. "We expect these problems will be surmounted by IMGs in a few years." Of greatest concern is that their grades are dependent on the impression they make on each evaluating person. The evaluating person is also likely to be biased by the fact that the examinee is an IMG who is trying to get into the United States and is a potential immigrant.

Several IMGs Association (AMA) have voiced similar views in many AMA meetings. Two other concerns expressed by some IMGs were as follows:

- Most of the research done by ECFMG prior to designing the CSA involved IMGs who were already residents of the United States. These foreign graduates are not really representative of most IMGs prior to entering a residency program in the United States. One colleague drew my attention to two papers, by Sutnick et al (JAMA 1993;270:1041–1045) and Ziv et al (Academic Medicine 1998;73:S83–S90), which discuss the design of the research done by ECGMG.
- Philadelphia is currently the only location at which the CSA is being given. This situation alone will eliminate many IMGs, who cannot afford to spend another $2000 to $3000 to come to the United States for the test.

POSSIBLE ADVANTAGES OF THE TEST

I spoke with several program directors of different residency programs around the United States, some of whom stated that it would be reassuring for them to know that a particular IMG had demonstrated competence in spoken English as well as clinical assessment of patients through the CSA. In addition, the test may help program directors appreciate some of the applicant's achievements as enumerated in his or her CV. Previously, the directors stated, they were often too preoccupied trying to ensure that an IMG had good basic skills to consider some of these other attributes.

WHO NEEDS TO TAKE THE CSA?

IMGs who did not fulfill all the conditions for ECFMG certification prior to July 1, 1998, will have to take the CSA before they can earn ECFMG certification. The conditions prior to July 1, 1998, were completion with a passing score of the USMLE steps 1 and 2, and the English proficiency test. Pre-July conditions apply to you if you took one of the exams prior to this date even though the result was received after June 30, 1998. If you did not pass all three exams before the cutoff date, you will now have to take the CSA to become ECFMG-certified.

Anyone who did not pass all three exams, including the USMLE 1 and 2, and the English exam, prior to June 30, 1998, must take the CSA to obtain ECFMG certification.

Let's consider another scenario, facing some IMGs. Suppose you had earned ECFMG certification in early 1998. You could not enter a residency program for 2 years after taking the English exam. So your certificate needs revalidation in, say, January 2000. Do you have to take only the English test again for revalidation or do you also have to take the CSA now? The answer is that the pre-July 1998 conditions still apply to you; you do not have to take the CSA.

VOLUNTARY TESTING

As I mentioned earlier in this chapter, some program directors have stated they have more trust in candidates who have taken the CSA. This has led some IMGs who were ECFMG-certified prior to July 1998 to conclude that taking the CSA may make them more competitive in the residency market. You are eligible to take the CSA even if you are already ECFMG-certified according to the old criteria. You can take CSA as long as you have not yet entered a residency program.

ELIGIBILITY CRITERIA FOR THE CSA

- You should be an IMG. That also applies to you if you are a U.S. citizen but graduated from a foreign medical school.
- You should have passed the USMLE 1 and 2, and the English proficiency test. That means you should have fulfilled all the eligibility criteria for those tests as enumerated in previous chapters.

APPLICATION PROCESS

APPLICATION FORM

The official four-part pink application form (Form 706) is inserted in the ECFMG information booklet. This form can be requested as explained in Chapter 4. The application form needs to be completed in the presence of the dean of your medical school. If that is not possible, you need to state the reason, as explained in Chapter 4. In that case, you should request the notary or the first-class magistrate to mail the form from his or her office. This form has to be accompanied by the CSA fee of U.S. $1200. As this test is given year-round, you can send the application form at any time. Once your completed form is received, ECFMG will evaluate your eligibility. If found eligible, you will receive notification of registration and information regarding scheduling of the test.

SCHEDULING THE TEST

Once you receive the notification from ECFMG, you must schedule a test date by calling 215-970-1982, Monday through Friday between 8 A.M. and 12 midnight Eastern standard time (EST). This must be made within 4 months of receipt of notification, and the test should be taken within 1 year of the notification. For example, suppose you receive the notification on January 1, 2001. You must call the number above to schedule the date before April 30, 2001, and the scheduled date for the test must be before December 31, 2001.

When you make this call, be ready to provide the following information:

1. The spelling of your name
2. Your ECFMG number
3. Your date of birth

You may not be able to schedule your first-choice date, so be sure to have more than one date in mind before you make this call. Keep in mind that once you have chosen a date, you are committed to taking the exam on that date. Your test will begin in the morning or afternoon on the scheduled date.

You may have to wait a considerable amount of time when you call before you reach a representative to help you with scheduling. This wait can be painfully expensive if you are making the call from outside the United States. If possible, you may wish to ask a dependable acquaintance in the United States to make the scheduling call for you. In this case, you should give the necessary information to the person making the call. Another way to schedule the CSA is through the Internet. If you have access to the Internet, this will probably be a much cheaper option than phoning directly.

However you choose to schedule the CSA, you will be committed to the date chosen and will be sent a written confirmation by regular mail. At this point, you cannot cancel or reschedule without forfeiting your fee. In some extraordinary circumstances, appeals can be made for an exception to this rule. The address for submission of appeal is as follows:

ECFMG
Attn: CSA Examination Exceptions Appeals
3624 Market Street
Philadelphia, PA 19104 USA

SCHEDULING STRATEGY

You will have to travel to the United States to take the exam. Quite naturally, many IMGs want to accomplish as much as possible while they are here to avoid the expense of another trip. The next steps to consider at this point are these:

- Waiting for the CSA result (6 to 8 weeks)
- Applying for a residency
- Scheduling and appearing for interviews
- Waiting for the match results

Schedule your visit carefully to allow you to accomplish as much as possible in the allotted time.

Taking these things into consideration, you should schedule the CSA around July or August. That way, you will have the results by September or October. You can apply for residency through Electronic Residency Application Service (ERAS) while you are waiting for the CSA results. Once you have the results, you should send updated information to ERAS advising that you have passed the CSA. In this way, you will still be in the United States when you are ready to schedule and appear for interviews, thus avoiding the hassle and expense of a return trip. You can also take step 3 of the USMLE at this point if you need to. I am suggesting this scenario on the assumption that you have a place to stay in the United States for about 6 months. In addition, you will also need to request a 6-month visa from the INS officials at the port of entry. You should be ready to explain why you want the visa for this length of time.

Some IMGs think it is necessary to be in the United States at the time the National Residency Matching Program (NRMP) match results are announced, which is in mid-March. The reasoning behind this is that if you do not match, it will be easier to look for a postmatch position while you are physically present in the United States. Of course, this means also you will have to be in the United States for another 3 months, which means you will have to extend your visitor's visa at least once.

TIMING THE APPLICATION FOR A VISA

There are three issues here: (1) You have to make arrangements to travel to the United States for the CSA; (2) anyone can be refused a visa; and (3) the CSA date, once set, cannot be changed. In view of this, you should apply for your visa before you send the application for CSA along with the fee of $1200. When obtaining the visa, you should request at least a 1-year tourist visa.

RECERTIFICATION

If you cannot join a residency program within 3 years of passing the CSA, you will have to have your ECFMG certificate revalidated by appearing for the CSA again. The process is exactly the same as for the initial CSA.

MAKING YOUR TRAVEL ARRANGEMENTS

As of the writing of this book, the CSA will be administered at only one location:

ECFMG
3624 Market Street
CSA Center, 3rd Floor
Philadelphia, PA 19104 USA

This is one of the main criticisms of the introduction of the exam. As previously noted, it is a widely held belief that many IMGs may not be able to take the test because they do not have enough money to travel to the United States.

Make any arrangements for travel within the United States before leaving your country.

Keep the following in mind when making your travel arrangements:

- Ask yourself if you have an acquaintance who might be ready to provide you with lodging for the duration of your stay. Look around at the people you know. Ask people. Sometimes even slight acquaintences can be very accommodating when they know your situation. Ideally this person should live as near to the CSA center as possible. If you are more than several hours away, you can make arrangements to arrive in Philadelphia the day before your scheduled exam date.
- Buy your airline tickets from a reputable agent in your own country.
- Obtain a visa for travel. (Refer to Chapter 2 for information about obtaining different types of visas.)
- Once you are in the United States, you can travel to Philadelphia by plane or Greyhound bus. Look for good deals on travel within the United States from your agent before leaving your home country. Check to see if you can buy Greyhound bus tickets in your country. Special discount rates are available for people coming to the United States on a visitor's visa; however, to obtain these rates you must purchase your tickets before arriving in the United States.

- Choose a place to stay in Philadelphia if you will need to arrive the day before the test. ECFMG may send you a list of hotels near the examination center where you can stay. This is a good place to start. It may also be worthwhile to do some research on your own to find a good, reasonably priced room. The Internet is another good resource. Or perhaps you know someone in the United States who is a member of the Automobile Association of America (known by its initials, AAA or "Triple A"). This is a motor club that helps its members plan their travels; this organization can supply members, free of charge, with guidebooks for specific locations that can help travelers choose a hotel that suits their budget. Yet another approach is to call the department of tourism in Philadelphia to ask them to mail you a list of hotels in the area. They should be able to supply this listing free of cost. It will include contact information and prices too.
- Be careful about what you eat. During this trip, it is better to stick to foods that you are familiar with. You can try the many available exotic foods on your next trip. For now, stick to the conventional. If you are fortunate enough to be able to stay with a person from your own country, you may be able to eat foods that you are used to.

CALLING ALL ENTREPRENEURS

The advent of the CSA has provided an opportunity for the entrepreneurial-minded. I have no doubt that such individuals will begin to offer packages to IMGs planning to come to the United States to take the exam. These packages should include:

- Good, reasonably priced travel arrangements
- Nice accommodations offering reasonable weekly or monthly prices
- Ethnic food

These requirements might be met, for example, by buying apartments or houses and hiring cooks to prepare particular ethnic foods. IMGs coming from different countries would no doubt feel reassured to deal with these agencies in their own countries and would appreciate the opportunity to purchase such a travel package rather than having to make their own plans.

CSA: THE EXAM

From an examinee's point of view, the CSA involves examining 11 standardized patients (SPs). Ten of these cases will be scored and one will be used for research. Each SP represents one test case. These cases reflect a mix of age, sex, and ethnic background, as well as acute, subacute, and chronic problems. They are designed to be characteristic of the types of cases you would be likely to encounter in clinics, doctor's offices, and emergency departments in the United States.

The CSA test cases represent the major clinical disciplines taught as part of the standard curriculum at medical schools accredited by the Liaison Committee on Medical Education (LCME) in the United States. These disciplines are as follows:

- Internal medicine
- Surgery
- Obstetrics and gynecology
- Pediatrics
- Psychiatry
- Family medicine

The test cases will not necessarily be divided equally among the different disciplines. Furthermore, it is usual for one case to test knowledge of different disciplines at the same time.

According to information provided by ECFMG, the selection of cases for each examinee is guided by specifications that define main content areas:

- Cardiovascular/respiratory
- Digestive/genitourinary
- Neurology/psychiatry
- Other (ear, eyes, nose, throat, musculoskeletal)

WHAT IS A "STANDARDIZED PATIENT" (SP)?

According to ECFMG, an SP is "a layperson trained to accurately and consistently portray a patient. SPs will respond to the questions from the examinees with answers appropriate to the case, and upon physical examination, will demonstrate appropriate physical findings." SPs are also trained to evaluate your performance from the following angles:

- ❑ Was an appropriate history taken?
- ❑ Was a proper physical exam performed?
- ❑ Were you able to communicate appropriately in English?
- ❑ How was your overall interaction with the patient?

I will discuss each of these areas in finer detail later in this chapter.

The SP is a new concept for most IMGs, and this component has given rise to many questions. Frequently asked questions and my responses follow:

SPs can be actors or patients with fixed signs who have trained to portray a patient.

Q: Who exactly is the SP?
A: Dr. Barrows has written in one of his papers (Academic Medicine 1993;68:443–451): "I reserve the term standardized patient as a broader umbrella for both simulated patients and actual patients who have been carefully coached to present their own illnesses in a standardized, unvarying way." It is very important to keep this definition in mind, as we all know that an ordinary person may not be able to simulate a hepatomegaly; however, a test case could be an actual patient with a large liver who is coached to act as an SP.

Q: The knowledge that the person I am examining is also in a way my examiner will make me nervous. What can I do to minimize this?
A: This feeling can make you behave abnormally. You have to treat these people like other patients you have seen during your training.

Q: SPs are laypeople who are trained to act as patients. Does this mean that examinees will not have to do a fundal exam because the SP cannot be "trained" to have fundal hemorrhages? Similarly, since a person cannot fake diminished pulses, does that mean that the examinee can get by with doing a very concise exam?
A: This approach will not work, for two reasons. First, SPs are trained to keep tabs on whether or not you perform the relevant parts of the exam and they evaluate you accordingly. Second, as noted by Dr. Barrow's definition, the SP can also be a person with physical findings who is trained to act as a standardized patient. Dr. Barrows, in the paper cited above, also gives a list of physical findings that can be simulated. I was astonished when I saw the list, which is reprinted in Table 7–1. Remember, more findings might have been added.

TABLE 7–1. Physical Signs That Can Be Simulated

Abdominal tenderness	Incoordination
Acute abdomen	Jaundice
Airway obstruction	Joint restriction
Anaphylactic shock	Joint warmth and redness
Aphasia	Kernig's sign
Asterixis	Kussmaul respiration
Athetosis	Lid lag
Beevor's sign	Muscle spasm
Brudzinski's sign	Muscle weakness
Carotid bruit	Nuchal rigidity
Cheyne-Stokes respiration	Parkinsonism
Chorea	Perspiration
Chronic obstructive airway disease	Photosensitivity
Coma/unresponsiveness	Pneumothorax
Confusion	Ptosis of the lid
Costovertebral-angle tenderness	Rebound tenderness (abdomen)
Decerebrate	Renal artery stenosis
Dilated pupil	Retardation
Doll's eye response	Rigidity
Dysarthria	Seizures
Extensor plantar response ("Babinski")	Sensory Loss
Facial paralysis	Shortness of breath
Gait abnormalities	Spasticity
Ataxia	"Stiff man" syndrome
Hemiparesis	Tachycardia (with some SPs)
Waddling	Tenderness/rigidity on palpation
Degenerative hip	Thyroid bruit
Hearing loss	Tremor
Hematemesis	Visual loss (central, peripheral)
Hyperactive tendon reflexes	Vomiting
Hyper/hypotension (rigged cuff)	Wheezing
Hypomania	

Source: Barrow HS. An overview of the uses of standardized patients for teaching and evaluating clinical skills. Acad Med 1993;68:443–451.

Q: I have heard that CSA has been implemented as a way of keeping IMGs out of the United States. Don't you think that the evaluators will be biased against the examinees? How can I possibly expect to pass in such a hostile atmosphere?
A: Let me suppose for a minute that everything you just said is absolutely correct. All human beings have some degree of bias. But failing all of the people who appear to take the CSA is simply not possible. *Somebody* has to pass. You can increase your chances of success by being professional and charming to the SPs. After all, they are human, too. What endears you to your real patients will also endear you to the SPs.

ABOUT THE EXAM

I will begin by enumerating the two major problems IMGs often have with the CSA.

1. The SPs are dressed in gowns. Many IMGs feel uncomfortable talking to and palpating, percussing, or auscultating a patient of the opposite sex under the gown. While you should be courteous to the patient and show proper respect for his or her dignity, you should not let unwarranted hesitation stand in the way of a proper examination.
2. Many IMGs get too worked up about nailing the right *diagnosis*. This is not the major requirement for passing. You will be graded more on your overall approach. For example, you may be able to correctly diagnose an exotic syndrome immediately upon walking into the room but may still fail for lack of a systematic approach.

The test should last about 5 to 8 hours. There will be two breaks and snacks will be provided during the breaks. Throughout the test you will be alone with the SPs (who are, as previously noted, evaluating you). You will be monitored through video cameras. The only way a physician examiner will know of your performance will be through the video film or your write-up of the cases. The ambience of the test is tailored to be very near that of an actual practice situation in the United States.

Before the test begins, you will be given an orientation to the room setup and test components. During the test, you will be expected to perform the steps described in Table 7–2. These steps are discussed in more detail later in the chapter.

TABLE 7–2. Steps in the Clinical Assessment of Each Case

1. Review the pertinent *patient information*, including vital signs, the reason for hospital visit, and the age and sex of the patient, located outside each patient's examination room.
2. Take a focused *history of the present illness;* that is, the history relevant to the chief complaint.
3. Obtain the *past medical history.*
4. Do a *review of systems;* that is, ask about any negative or positive history pertaining to each major system (e.g., cardiovascular, respiratory, etc.) as relevant to the patient's main complaint.
5. Ask about *medications, allergies, dietary history, and immunizations.*
6. If the patient is female, take a *menstrual and obstetrical history.*
7. Obtain a *family history.*
8. Obtain a *social history,* including addictions, history of smoking or drinking, occupation, where and with whom the patient stays, marital status.
9. Perform the *relevant physical examination.*
10. *Discuss your initial diagnostic impression* and your workup plan with the patient. You should be ready to answer any questions the SP may ask.

    Note: These steps must be completed within 15 minutes. You will be given a warning when only 5 minutes are left. At the expiration of this time or whenever you have finished, you should thank the patient and leave the room. Once you leave the room, you cannot reenter it, so you should be sure you have completed all of the appropriate steps. You will have blank sheets of paper on which to take notes while you are talking to the patient so that you do not forget the information later.
11. *Write up* the patient information. After you leave the room, you will have 10 minutes to write up the information you have obtained in well-organized and legible form. This write-up should include the differential diagnoses up to a maximum of five, as well as the workup plan.

    A similar routine will need to be followed for all 11 patients.

THINGS NOT TO DO WHILE WORKING ON EACH CASE

Do not perform rectal, pelvic, or genital examinations or a female breast exam. If you think it is important for a particular case, suggest the pertinent exam as part of your workup. Do not include treatment, consultations, or referrals in your workup plan. Do not order a battery of tests; be specific in ordering tests. Also, do not order the most expensive test for each case; try to order tests that will point you in the right direction. According to ECFMG, the following standard multiple-component tests can be ordered:

- Complete blood count (CBC)
- Urinalysis
- Electrolytes
- Arterial blood gases

SCORING COMPONENTS

The following components are evaluated for each examinee:

1. The ability to elicit an appropriate history and perform the relevant physical exam
2. The ability to write a pertinent patient note
3. The quality of interpersonal skills, including interviewing skills
4. The clarity of spoken English

Items 1 and 2 are combined under the heading of integrated clinical encounter (ICE); items 3 and 4 are bunched under the communication (COM) score by the ECFMG.

ON THE DAY OF THE EXAM

You should make arrangements to reach the examination center on time. Pay particular attention to the following aspects:

- You will not be provided with closed lockers, so do not take any valuables to the examination hall. Be sure to place your passport in a secure spot with your belongings.
- Dress professionally. Wear a clean well-ironed white coat. This may have your name embroidered on left side above the pocket area.
- Listen carefully during the orientation session. Figures 7–1, 7–2, and 7–3 illustrate the features of a prototypical patient examination room. The examination rooms used for the test will not be exact replicas of that shown in the photographs. Be sure you know how to use the ophthalmoscope and the otoscope, and anything else in the room. Also know how to extend the examination table, and how to use it to prop up the patient. If in doubt, ask during the orientation.

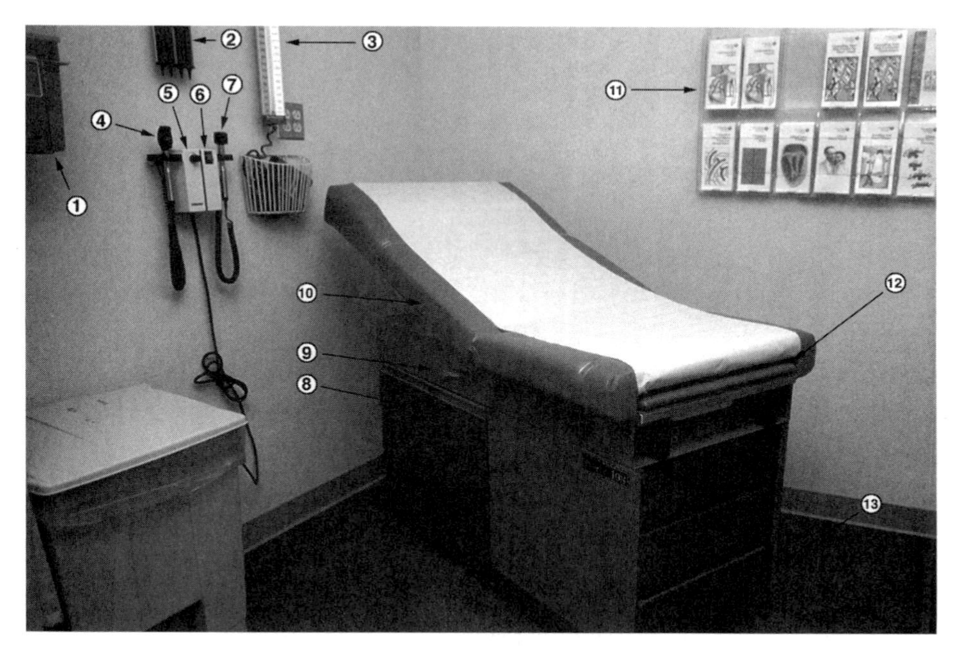

FIGURE 7–1. (1) Box for disposal of sharp objects such as needles. (2) Disposable ear pieces for an otoscope. (3) Blood pressure apparatus. (4) Ophthalmoscope that can be taken off the clip. (5) Button to adjust the intensity of light in an ophthalmoscope or otoscope. (6) Switch for power. (7) Otoscope. (8) Shelf for fresh gowns, sheets, and so forth. (9) Knob to adjust the head of the table. (10) Adjustable head end of the table. (11) Reading material for patients. (12) Table extension, which should be pulled out once the patient lies down so that his or her legs can rest there. (13) Table extension that can be pulled out and used as a step when the patients get onto and off the examination table.

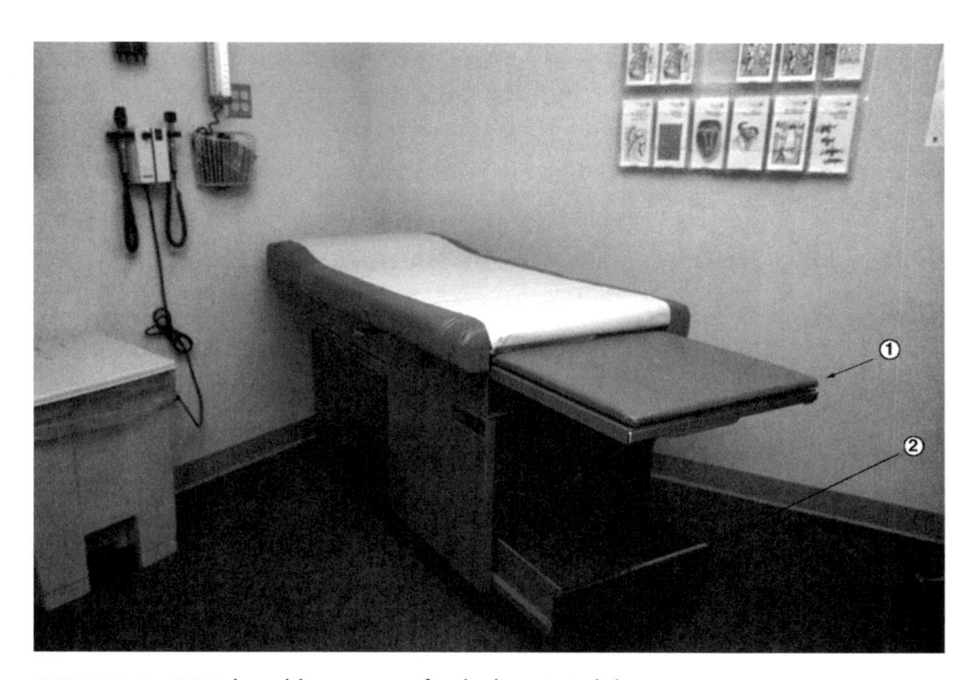

FIGURE 7–2. (1) Adjustable extension for the legs. (2) Sliding step.

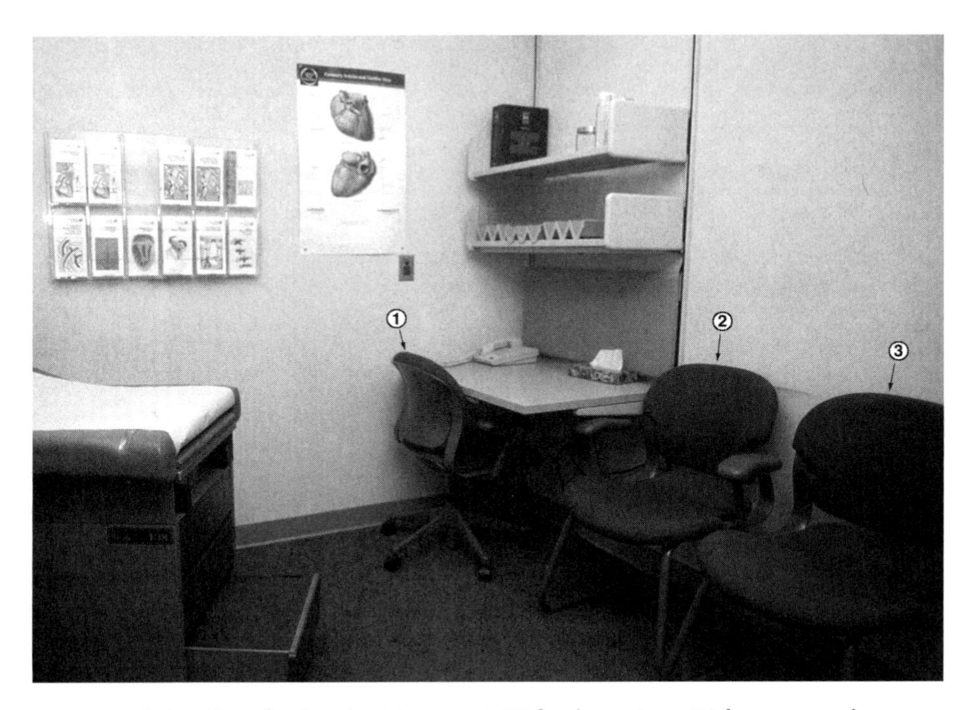

FIGURE 7–3 (1) Chair for the physician (you,) (2) for the patient, (3) for anyone else.

- Do not discuss the SPs with other candidates. Do not communicate in any language other than in English. When in doubt, assume that someone is watching you. In all probability, nothing you say or do will escape the watchful eyes of the test administrators and their video cameras.

STEP-BY-STEP APPROACH TO DOING WELL ON THE CSA

STEP 1: HOW TO BEGIN

When allowed to start with a case, begin by reading the patient information posted on the doorway. Similar information will also be available in the room. You will have some blank sheets on which to take notes. Special attention should be given to the patient's name and chief complaint.

Enter the room with a relaxed and confident manner. Be seated and see that the SP is comfortable in his or her seat. Address the SP as Mr. or Ms. followed by the last name and introduce yourself as Dr. followed by your last name. As in a real practice situation in the United States, you may not be sure whether a female patient is married. So it is often best to address the patient as "Ms." rather than debating about whether to use "Mrs." or "Miss." From this point on in the chapter, I will refer to the SPs as patients, as that is how I would like you to think about them. Repeat the chief complaint as written on the doorway sheet and ask for permission to obtain a history and perform a physical examination of the patient. The conversation could go something like this: "Mr. Smith, I am Dr. Sanchez. I understand you are here because of pain in your abdomen. Can we talk about your problem in greater detail?"

STEP 2: HISTORY OF PRESENT ILLNESS

Tell the patient that you will be taking notes on a piece of paper while talking to him or her. In real life, this keeps the patient informed of everything you are doing. At this stage, you should talk about the patient's chief complaint. This is called the history of present illness. Let the patient explain the problem. Show interest in the problem, and listen carefully. Curb the tendency to interrupt while the patient is talking. This is a natural response when you are rushed for time, as here, where you have only 15 minutes for each case. You can, however, use good interviewing skills to keep the patient focused on the main problem. Your goal is to acquire data that will help you make a diagnosis based on the history. This part of the history will also direct you toward things to look for in the physical exam. As an example, if a patient presents with chest pain, you need to ask about the characteristics of the pain that will likely help you in differentiating between different causes of chest pain. You want to develop a good rapport with the patient and to acquire all the relevant data while being careful not to brush aside the patient's concerns thoughtlessly. If you do not understand a certain part of the patient's conversation, excuse yourself and request further clarification.

Apart from these suggestions, the real secret to taking a pertinent history and performing a physical examination is using analytical acumen based on the knowledge you have acquired by examining other patients during your training.

After acquiring data about the present illness, if time permits, tell the patient that you will summarize the information and ask the patient to correct you if you are wrong. This reassures the patient that he or she conveyed all the relevant points to you.

STEP 3: PAST MEDICAL HISTORY

Ask about any history of past medical problems. Let the patient volunteer information; then ask the questions regarding the past medical history that are relevant to the case.

STEP 4: REVIEW OF SYSTEMS (ROS)

The ROS involves reviewing each major body system one at a time to see whether any special history in relation to that system needs to be elicited. This needs to be decided on the basis of the patient's presenting complaint and your possible diagnosis. As an example, if the patient has arthritis, you may want to ask about urethral discharge in the genitourinary system, painful eye in HEENT (head, eye, ear, nose, throat), and so on. The ROS need not be a laundry list of all the symptoms known to humankind.

STEP 5: MEDICATIONS, ALLERGIES, DIETARY HISTORY

Medications

Ask what medications the patient is taking. In the United States most patients are well aware of the medications they are taking, and there are only a few medications that can be bought without a doctor's prescription. These nonprescription medications are called over-the-counter (OTC) drugs. It is important to ask the patient specifically if he or she is taking any OTC drugs, because some patients may not consider these to be medications and may forget to mention them. Obtaining such information is important, for example, in the case of a patient with a bleeding ulcer who regularly takes aspirin, an OTC drug.

Allergies

Ask about any medications the patient is allergic to. Whenever an allergy is reported, ask about the nature of the allergic reaction. This is important because sometimes the patient may link unrelated symptoms with the administration of a medicine. This information helps keep open the option of using the same medicine in the future.

Diet

Ask if the patient follows a special diet; examples include fad diets, low-sodium diet, low-fluid diet, renal diet, and so on.

STEP 6: MENSTRUAL AND OBSTETRICAL HISTORY

Obtain a menstrual history from female patients. This is helpful if you want to order radiological tests. Sometimes this information may clinch a diagnosis; for example, pain in the abdomen of a woman who missed her last period will point you toward ectopic pregnancy. Do not presume that a female patient cannot have children or pregnancy because she looks young or is not married. Do not prejudge anything. Follow a systematic approach.

STEP 7: FAMILY HISTORY

Obtain a history of any medical problems in the family that are likely to be relevant to the present problem. As a general rule, it is a better idea to ask if any members of the patient's family have any significant medical problems. This segment may require some tact on your part, for instance, if patient starts to tell you a story about his grandma's dentures. In such a situation, just say politely, "That's okay Mr. Joel, that may not have any bearing on your present problem."

STEP 8: SOCIAL HISTORY

The following elements are important aspects of the social history:

- Abuse of illicit drugs.
- Smoking and drinking alcohol.
- Occupational history.
- Patient's social support system.
- Marital status. Do not presume that a person is married just because he or she has children.
- Sexual preferences. If you feel uncomfortable asking a question, you might say something like, "Excuse me, Mr./Ms.___, I hope you do not mind me asking, but have you ever felt sexually aroused by a person of the same sex?" Although this can be an uncomfortable question to ask, you have to be able to demonstrate that you can elicit a relevant history without letting personal hesitation get in your way.
- Preventive health measures.

You may be unfamiliar with some aspects of the social history as obtained in the United States.

Additional information on some of the areas is provided in Chapter 12.

STEP 9: RELEVANT PHYSICAL EXAMINATION

I will explain the techniques and steps of the physical exam in more detail in Chapter 12. Here I wish to focus on a few things that are most relevant to the CSA examination.

- After you have finished taking the history, ask the patient's permission to examine him or her. If the patient is not wearing a gown, ask the patient to take off his or her top and wear a gown with the front side (toward the chest) open. Give the patient a gown and walk out of the room while he or she is changing. Where are the gowns kept? That should be another question you ask during the orientation. Also ask the person giving the orientation if the patients will already be wearing gowns when you see them.
- Next, ask the patient to lie down on the examination table. Offer your hand if the patient is having difficulty moving to or getting onto the table. Help the patient into a comfortable position.
- You are now ready to begin the examination. Wash your hands before and after examining the patient. Be sure your hands are not too cold when you begin the examination.
- Present a comfortably confident demeanor. Be considerate of the patient. Let the patient know what you will be doing before each part of the exam. For example, say you are going to auscultate the heart before you slide your stethoscope under the patient's gown. Tell the patient you are going to examine the abdomen before doing so. Do not perform those parts of examination enumerated earlier in this chapter. By the same token, do not let unnecessary cautiousness prevent you from performing a thorough exam. I am sure I am not telling you anything that is new to you. But it is important to keep focused as you try to complete the necessary actions in the 15 minutes allotted to each case.
- Offer to assist the patient off the table.
- Keep the atmosphere light, without straining to be humorous.

STEP 10: DISCUSSION WITH THE PATIENT

After completing the history and physical exam, you need to sit down with the patient to explain your initial impression about his or her problem. This can be especially problematic when you are trying to complete all of the steps in a fixed time period. You will have to pace yourself during the history and physical exam so you have a few minutes at the end of each session for this step. As with any other step, you are scored on this aspect too.

My research has turned up several issues that IMGs should be aware of, as follows:

- You do not have to act like you know everything about the patient's problem. You do not have to offer one crisp answer to all the patient's problems. Tell the patient about various possibilities you are considering, and state what you are going to do to prove or disprove them. Do not feel pressured to present a picture of yourself as a know-it-all genius. If the patient asks a question, try to answer it in the best way possible on the basis of your knowledge. If you are not sure, concede ignorance and offer to find the answer at a later date.
- Be prepared to explain various things in a layperson's language. For example, if you are ordering a CT scan, on inquiry from the patient, you may have to say something like, "You will be put on a table and a tube around your head will take various pictures. . . ."
- Do not give false reassurance. Whatever you say should be based on facts.

You must train yourself to be able to discuss the patient's condition with him or her. "Don't worry, I will take care of everything" is not an acceptable approach.

It may be helpful here to review a few of the situations I have come across that may be simulated in the CSA.

1. Do not let your personal biases dictate the way you advise the patient. Some examples include lashing out at a patient bringing up the question of abortion because you hold staunch pro-life opinions, or disparaging alternative medicine because you think it is unscientific.
2. If a patient becomes angry at something you say, give your point of view on why you said what you said. Do not let the patient throw you off balance. An angry patient may be a dramatic sight, especially to IMGs from countries where doctors are virtually idolized.
3. Be respectful of the patient's wishes. If he or she refuses to follow your request at any point during the history or physical examination, politely explain why that part is important and withdraw.
4. Many patients in the United States obtain information on their condition from publications or the Internet. These patients are often quite savvy about their condition. Refer to Chapter 13 for further discussion.

STEP 11: WRITING IT DOWN

After you exit the patient's room, you will be given 10 minutes to write up the history (including various aspects discussed above), physical exam, differential diagnosis, and suggested diagnostic workup on the sheet provided. I cannot emphasize too strongly that this write-up must be legible, because this is a critical component on which you will be evaluated.

Apart from this, you need to understand the functions served by a doctor's note in real-life situations:

- Providing care to a patient involves teamwork. The various team players include nurses, pharmacists, other physicians, consultants, and other ancillary staff. Your note should reflect what you think about the patient's problem and the rationale behind your thought process. Depending on where you belong in the given team structure, a well-organized note from you will help other members of your team perform better.
- Your own notes should be able to give you a clear picture of your own thought process if you have to go back to them after a significant period of time has passed.

The ways to achieve these goals are as follows:

- Write in a well-organized fashion. The note should be a written account of your thinking process. For example, if a patient has a painful abdomen, your note should specify the site and radiation of pain, any relation to meals, any bowel or bladder trouble, and so on. That will show you were thinking of various causes of abdominal pain and you systematically ruled them in or out. Similarly, the note should provide a specific account listing of the presence or absence of findings such as tenderness, guarding, rebound, or organomegaly.
- If you need to correct something after writing, simply run a line through it and write the word "error" under or on top of the scratched out part. That shows that you purposefully intended to change that part.

USE OF ABBREVIATIONS

All of us have used certain abbreviations in writing up our clinical notes. Some are internationally recognized but the majority happen to be a local institutional phenomenon. ECFMG provides a list of abbreviations that you are allowed to use in the write-ups for the CSA. This list will be available to you on-site when you take the exam. It is reprinted in Table 7–3.

TABLE 7–3. List of Approved Abbreviations for Use in the CSA

Abbreviation	Meaning
Units of Measure	
kg	kilogram
g	gram
mg	milligram
μg	microgram
lbs	pounds
oz	ounce
m	meter
cm	centimeter
min	minute
hr	hour
C	Centigrade
F	Fahrenheit
Vital Signs	
BP	blood pressure
P	pulse
R	respirations
T	temperature
Routes of Drug Administration	
IM	intramuscularly
IV	intravenously
po	orally
General Medical Terms	
AIDS	acquired immunodeficiency syndrome
AP	anteroposterior
BUN	blood urea nitrogen
CABG	coronary artery bypass grafting
CBC	complete blood count
CCU	cardiac care unit
CHF	congestive heart failure
COPD	chronic obstructive pulmonary disease
CPR	cardiopulmonary resuscitation
CT	computerized tomography
CVA or TIA	cerebrovascular or transient ischemic accident
CVP	central venous pressure
DTR	deep tendon reflexes
ECG	electrocardiogram
ED	emergency department
EMT	emergency medical technician
ENT	ears, nose, and throat
EOM	extraocular muscles
HEENT	head, eyes, ears, nose, and throat
HIV	human immunodeficiency virus
HPF	high power field
JVD	jugular venous distention
KUB	kidney, ureter, and bladder
LMP	last menstrual period
LP	lumbar puncture
MI	myocardial infarction
MVA	motor vehicle accident
NIDDM	noninsulin-dependent diabetes mellitus
NKA	no known allergies
NKDA	no known drug allergy
NL	normal limits
NSR	normal sinus rhythm
PA	posteroanterior
PERLA	pupils equal, reactive to light and accommodation
PT	prothrombin time
PTT	partial thromboplastin time

TABLE 7–3. List of Approved Abbreviations for Use in the CSA *(Continued)*

RBC	red blood cells
URI	upper respiratory tract infection
WBC	white blood cells
WNL	within normal limits
Commonly Used Abbreviations in the Patient Note	
yo	year-old
m	male
f	female
b	black
w	white
l	left
r	right
hx	history
c/o	complaining of
h/o	history of
DM	diabetes mellitus
HTN	hypertension
GI	gastrointestinal
FH	family history
SH	social history
cig	cigarettes
ETOH	alcohol
GU	genitourinary
Abd	abdomen
Ext	extremities
Neuro	neurological
U/A	urinalysis
CXR	chest X-ray
MRI	magnetic resonance imaging

Source: ECFMG website at *www.ecfmg.org*.

The Test of Spoken English (TSE) is not required for ECFMG certification, but it may be a useful evaluation tool for those concerned about their command of English.

NOT SURE OF YOUR COMMAND OF ENGLISH?

I have met several IMGs living outside the United States who felt they were prepared to take the CSA but were unsure whether their ability to speak English was acceptable. To get an objective evaluation of your spoken English ability, you can take the Test of Spoken English (TSE), which is administered by TOEFL. This is not a requirement for ECFMG certification. An information bulletin about the test can be ordered in the following ways:

- Online by going to *www.toefl.com.*
- By writing to:
  TOEFL/TSE Services
  P.O. Box 6151
  Princeton, NJ USA 08541-6151
- By calling 609-771-7100

According to information provided by ECFMG, studies have revealed that candidates who obtained a score of 35 or lower on the TSE are unlikely to demonstrate the level of spoken English proficiency required to pass the CSA.

WHAT IF I FAIL THE CSA?

Candidates who fail the CSA will have to reapply to take the exam. The repeat test cannot be rescheduled until 3 months after a failure.

CHAPTER 8

USMLE Step 3

The USMLE step 3 must be taken by all IMGs who want to practice as physicians in the United States. This exam is not a requirement for entry into a residency program in the United States, and most IMGs, as well as American graduates take this exam toward the end of their first year of residency training. However, some IMGs arrange to take the exam even before starting their residency for following reasons:

- The USMLE 3 must be taken before IMGs can get an H-1 visa for residency training.
- Some IMGs think that taking the USMLE 3, in addition to satisfying other requirements for entry into a residency program, may improve their chances of getting into the program.

REGISTRATION

The registration requirements for the USMLE 3 are decided by each individual state. For general information on medical licensure and step 3, contact the Federation of State Medical Boards (FSMB). Their postal address is:

FSMB
400 Fuller Wiser Road, Suite 300
Euless, TX 76039-3855
Tel: 817-571-2949

The basic requirement for all IMGs is the possession of an ECFMG certificate issued prior to the published deadline date for the exam. Several states allow physicians to take the USMLE 3 before starting a residency program. These are listed in Table 8–1.

TABLE 8–1. States that Do Not Require Residency Training Before Taking the USMLE 3

California	Connecticut	Maryland
Nevada	New York	Puerto Rico
South Dakota	Tennessee	West Virginia

Note: Nebraska and Utah do not require any postgraduate training to sit for the USMLE 3, but they require that IMGs have an ECFMG certificate validated "indefinitely" prior to taking the USMLE 3. The ECFMG certificate cannot be validated indefinitely unless one enters an accredited residency program.
Source: FSMB at *www.fsmb.org*.

According to the FSMB, the application material for the USMLE 3 in following states can be obtained by calling FSMB at 817-868-4000.

Alaska	Mississippi
Arizona	Nebraska
Arkansas	Nevada
Colorado	New Hampshire
Connecticut	Oregon
Delaware	Rhode Island
Hawaii	South Dakota
Iowa	Tennessee
Maine	Vermont
Michigan	Washington
Minnesota	Wyoming

This information may change from time to time. To obtain the application material from states other than those above you should call the individual state medical boards. The full address and telephone numbers can be obtained from the FSMB Website at *www.usmle.org/99boi/FSMB.htm*.

Useful information enumerating state licensing board requirements for IMGs is also available on the American Medical Association (AMA) Website at *www.ama-assn.org*. You should go to the "IMG quick fact" section. This page provides information regarding different requirements for individual states in a tabulated format. You should contact the individual state boards for the latest requirements. This page also gives contact telephone numbers for all state boards.

Worth mentioning here (source *www.ama-assn.org*) is that different states have different requirements as they apply to persons on the "fifth pathway." The fifth pathway is available to persons studying abroad who have:

1. Completed their premedical work in a U.S.-accredited college equivalent to matriculation in an accredited U.S. medical school
2. Studied in a foreign medical school listed in the WHO *World Directory of Medical Schools*
3. Satisfied all requirements for admission to practice except internship or social service in a foreign country

IMGs holding a fifth pathway but not holding an ECFMG certificate can be admitted to the licensing exam in all states except Alabama, Alaska, Arkansas, Indiana, Michigan, Tennessee, Texas, and Vermont.

SCHEDULING

When you receive the application material from the appropriate state board, complete it and send it back to the given address along with the required documents and appropriate fee. As of fall 1999, the USMLE 3 has become computer based. This change will affect the scheduling process somewhat, as for steps 1 and 2, described earlier in Chapters 4 and 5. Once the state board is satisfied that you are eligible to take the exam, you will receive a scheduling permit. The permit will specify a 90-day period during which you must take the test. You should call a Sylvan center directly after receiving the permit to set up an appointment for the exam.

The change to computer-based testing (CBT) is recent and the scheduling instructions and exam pattern may change during this initial period. Read the information sent to you at the time of registration carefully.

According to the FSMB, step 3 can be rescheduled with a minimum of 5 days' advance notice. The cutoff time is noon Eastern Standard Time (EST; i.e., New York time). If an exam is rescheduled with less than 5 days' notice, the Sylvan center will charge a rescheduling fee.

COMPUTER-BASED TESTING

The initial formalities on the day of exam should be same as those for the USMLE 1 and 2. The total duration of the exam is 16 hours over 2 days, with 8 hours each day. On the first day, a 15-minute orientation and tutorial are given, followed by four blocks of test items. Each block contains 25 to 50 questions. The time provided ranges from 30 to 60 minutes. There is midday lunch break, with three or four blocks in the afternoon. The second day starts with an orientation to the Primum CCS software. The test items on this day include three blocks of case simulation (each with two or four cases) and an additional three or four blocks of multiple-choice questions.

The new computer-based testing format of the USMLE 3 will bring in two unique features: computer-based, case simulation (CCS) and computer-adaptive sequential testing (CAST).

COMPUTER-BASED CASE SIMULATION (CCS)

According to the FSMB, CCS is a computer-based interactive test format that allows the examinee to care for a simulated patient. You may request information from the history and physical examination, order laboratory studies, and start medications or therapies. When you do not wish to do anything more, you can reevaluate the patient by clicking on the clock icon to advance the time. The patient's condition will be shown to have changed over time. You may view patient charts with updated information such as lab results, vital signs, and progress and nurse's notes. Your actions will be compared to those of experts. You will be judged on the basis of the sequence and timing of the steps taken as well as whether the patient's condition was jeopardized as a result of your actions or failure to act.

COMPUTER-ADAPTIVE SEQUENTIAL TESTING (CAST)

In CAST, the computer periodically calculates the examinee's performance measure, then selects the following test materials to most efficiently meet the measurement objectives of the test. This feature will be introduced on a small section of the examination initially as CBT is introduced in the USMLE 3.

"COMPUTERESE"

As noted in Chapters 4 and 5 on USMLE 1 and 2, you should be familiar with computers before you even think of taking the USMLE 3. You must be thoroughly familiar with the Primum software as well. A CD-Rom containing this software will be sent to all registrants with the application package. A computer with a CD drive and an audio system is required to use this CD.

ABOUT THE EXAM

According to the USMLE, "step 3 assesses whether an examinee can apply the medical knowledge and understanding of biomedical and clinical science considered essential for the unsupervised practice of medicine, with special emphasis on patient management in ambulatory settings."

Examinees are asked questions that presume they are primary care physicians practicing medicine independently and capable of taking care of patients in different care settings. It is therefore very important that IMGs understand the practice style of a primary care physician in the United States.

PRACTICE PARAPHERNALIA

Visualize yourself in the ambience of a practice setting for a general practitioner in the United States.

1. In the United States, physicians are most likely to encounter patients in the following settings: office, in-patient facilities, emergency department, on the phone, or in a satellite health center.
   a. Office: This is the setting where patients are seen by appointments. Such patients are usually known to the doctor and are coming in for regularly scheduled visits. Group practice is a popular mode of practice in the United States in which several doctors get together and work in a group. Different members of the group are associates. When one of the associates goes on vacation, another doctor in the group "covers" by seeing his or her patients. The covering doctor has access to the charts of these patients. The charts of active patients are kept on the office premises. As a physician in this setting, you can admit patients from the office. You also have access to the full range of laboratory and radiological services for the patients seen in the office setting.
   b. In-patient facilities: As a generalist, you would admit patients to the hospital and also take care of them. Apart from typical patients admitted to the wards, you might also see patients in the following settings:
      - Children's and women's services
      - Critical care. A critical care specialist deals with more intricate details. But you will follow some of your patients in this setting.
      - Postoperative follow-up
      - Psychiatric unit
      - Nursing home: This is the term commonly used to refer to facilities designed for patients who require long-term care. These are patients who cannot take care of themselves owing to a physical or mental infirmity. The health care

demands of these patients are typically beyond the capacity of their family members. A majority of these patients are elderly people who may be sent to a nursing home for the remainder of their lives. Others may return to the community after an acute health crisis is over or when their social situation changes.

c. Emergency department (ED): Patients in this setting require urgent attention. Most of these patients would be new to you; however, you might ask some of your regular patients to go to the ED on the basis of complaints conveyed to you over the phone.

d. Phone contact: Sometimes a physician's regular patients will phone the office to clarify the dosage of a medicine or to report a new symptom. In these cases, you would have to take a focussed history over the phone to decide about the possible reason for the symptoms. Most important, you would need to be able to decide if the patient needed to be seen right away. The patient might get in touch with you directly or talk to your office assistant and leave a message. These phone calls could come in during regular office hours or after hours. On days when you were on call in a group practice, you might get calls from your associates' patients who might not be known to you. You would need to be able to give them advice on the basis of information acquired over the phone, as well as to tell them if they needed to see their doctor any earlier than their scheduled visit in view of the symptoms reported to you. If a patient needed emergency care, you would advise him or her to go to the ED.

e. Satellite health center: For the purpose of the examination, this setting is defined by the USMLE as a "community-based health facility where patients seeking both routine and urgent care are encountered. Students from a nearby small university use this setting as a student health service. Several industrial parks and local small businesses send employees with on-the-job injuries and for the employee health screening. Usually you are seeing the patients for the first time. There is capability for x-ray films, but CT and MRI must be arranged at the hospital."

2. After a patient is discharged from the hospital, he or she may go to one of the following settings: home, nursing home, or rehabilitation centers. Terminally ill patients may also be referred for hospice care.
   a. Rehabilitation center: Patients are sometimes discharged to an in-patient rehabilitation center. Such centers may specialize in providing one type of care; for example, assisting patients to overcome a substance abuse problem, recover from a brain injury, or improve their physical functioning.
   b. Hospice: The term "hospice" refers to a mode of management rather than a place where care is provided. This type of care can be provided at the patient's home or in a separate facility. Hospice care is designed for the people whose life expectancy is less than 6 months. The focus of care is palliative (focused on comfort measures) rather than curative.

   You would seek the help of a social worker to arrange discharge of any patient needing special arrangements.
3. You may need to put extra effort toward communicating well with both patients and their relatives.
4. Physicians in practice in the United States interact with many other personnel in various settings. You should be familiar with the roles of the following individuals.
   a. Consultants: These are your colleagues in other specialties or subspecialties. You should know when to refer a patient to a specialist.
   b. Secretaries or clerks: These are the people working on the ward floor. The secretary or clerk will take down the orders you write and enter them into the computer. These individuals do not have a medical background, but they know what constitutes a properly written order. Always write orders with clear-cut instructions. The medication order should include the dose, frequency, time (if applicable), and route of administration. The lab orders or orders for diagnostic studies should clearly define when they need to be done.
   c. Nurses: All of the members of health care team are working for the well-being of the patient. Always listen to the nurses' suggestions with an open mind.

d. Medical assistants: These are the people who help you in the office. They take calls from patients who wish to schedule appointments. They are the first contact for people coming to the office. The medical assistant shows the patient to an examination room, takes the vital signs, and talks with the patient about any special concerns before you see the patient. The assistant will also set up the appointments for any studies you order. He or she will take calls from patients who have concerns or problems. If the assistant cannot handle the patient's problem, he or she will have you speak with the patient. Clinic assistants can help you obtain old records of a patient. If the records need to be requested from another hospital, the patient must sign a "release of information" form, which authorizes your office to acquire the information. A patient's health record is a patient's personal property and it should not be released to anyone (even a family member) without the patient's consent.

e. ED personnel: This includes the ED doctors and their staff. Most patients going to the ED will be seen and evaluated by these individuals. This includes the patients you refer as well as those who seek care on their own. ED personnel will do a brief history and physical, order lab and radiology tests, take care of emergent issues, and then call you. You will then have to decide about the patient's treatment course on the basis of the information provided by the ED doctors.

You will have access to other services including rape/crisis intervention, family support, and security services backed by the local police. Become familiar with the role of these services.

PASS/FAIL STATISTICS

The pass/fail statistics for IMGs taking the USMLE 3 are shown in Table 8–2.

STEP 3: THE EXAM

The USMLE 3 is designed along two axes, namely, clinical encounter and physician tasks.

CLINICAL ENCOUNTER FRAMES

There are three different categories, as described below.

TABLE 8–2. Number of Enrollees Tested and Percent Passing the USMLE Step 3 in 1998

	May 1998		December 1998		1998 Total	
Registrants	No. Tested	% Passing	No. Tested	% Passing	No. Tested	% Passing
Total U.S./Canadian graduates	10,214	93	7,541	92	17,755	93
IMGs						
First-time takers	3,620	59	4,588	54	8,208	56
Repeaters	2,174	45	2,689	38	4,863	41
Total IMGs	5,794	54	7,277	48	13,071	51

Source: National Board of Medical Examiners.

Category I

The patients included in this frame are those who are seen for the first time on an outpatient basis. This could also include the patient whose history is available but who comes in with a new complaint. The problems could be the following:

- Acute with a limited course (e.g., cystitis, sore throat, etc.)
- Behavioral–emotional
- Initial presentations of chronic problems

The objective of the test items belonging to this category is to evaluate your ability to gather data and initiate initial clinical intervention. You may have to carry out an urgent intervention if the circumstances so demand.

Category II

Continuing management of previously diagnosed patients in the ambulatory setting characterizes the encounters in this frame. The examples might include:

- The patient with a known history of coronary artery disease who comes for a follow up examination. You should be able to take care of any new complaints as well as think of modifying risk factors such as cholesterol, smoking, and so on.
- The patient with chronic obstructive pulmonary disease (COPD) who comes to you with increasing shortness of breath. You should look for any exacerbating factors. You should also use this visit

as an opportunity to review whether the patient needs any preventive measures for overall well-being. These steps may not have any relation to the chief complaint. You should also suggest any age- and condition-appropriate screening tests.

- One of your patients who has been diagnosed with cancer and is receiving chemotherapy and who comes to you for an outpatient visit. You should be able to evaluate new complaints in light of the side effects of chemotherapy as well as possible progression of the disease. You may also be asked questions such as, "How much longer do I have to live, doctor?" You should be able to give a truthful answer in the most humane way possible.

This category also includes patient encounters characterized by complications or exacerbation of chronic conditions. These encounters may occur in the hospital setting. As an example, one of your patients with hypertension who presents with a stroke; a patient with diabetes mellitus who suffers a myocardial infarction.

The questions items included in this category emphasize the following abilities:

- The ability to manage and anticipate new problems in an existing condition. For this, you should be aware of the patient's life history, the projected course of the condition as well as signs and accompaniments to various chronic problems. This knowledge should also give you the ability to assess the prognosis of a given condition.
- The ability to assess the severity of any problem.
- The ability to follow patients with various chronic diseases on a long-term basis. This means being on the lookout for any complications of the patient's chronic and incurable medical condition, and maintaining the status quo. While doing this, you are also expected to assess the overall mental and physical well-being of your patients.

Category III

These encounters take place in the ED setting. The patient comes to you with life-threatening problems, and you have to make a quick assessment and initiate management. Occasionally, this may happen in the setting of a patient already in the hospital whose condition deteriorates suddenly. Here, you should be able to analyze the situation in view of the history of chronic disease.

The question items included in this category evaluate your ability to quickly assess patients and initiate appropriate management.

PHYSICIAN TASKS

This is the second axis along which the exam is designed. You are evaluated on various aspects that are essential to providing effective and appropriate medical care in the primary care setting.

- You should be able to make decisions on the basis of the history and physical examination data. You should be able to interpret the patient's comments.
- You should be able to choose the most effective, educated, and cost-effective way of diagnosing a condition with adequate certainty. You should also know when not to schedule a test. This could be either when you are certain of the diagnosis on the basis of the history and physical exam or your line of management is not going to change on the basis of the test results.
- You should be able to formulate the most likely diagnosis.
- You should be able to assess the severity of the patient's condition. Based on this knowledge, you should be able to take a realistic decision about whether you need to treat the patient more aggressively or instead adopt a palliative approach.
- Apart from taking care of patients and treating various diseases, you should also focus on health maintenance. You should be aware of common legal and ethical issues you are likely to encounter in the course of your practice as a physician. These issues will be explained in Chapter 13.

The rough percentage of test items belonging to different categories is shown in Table 8–3.

CCS: AN INTRODUCTION

As previously mentioned, this is a new feature of the USMLE 3. Computer-based case simulation (CCS) consists of several cases, each of which provides an interactive simulation of a patient care environment. The description of the practice environment in the United States earlier in this chapter should help you feel more comfortable in

TABLE 8–3. Approved Step 3 Blueprint

	Clinical Encounter Frames			
Physician Tasks	**Initial Workup 1**	**Continued Care 2**	**Emergency 3**	**TOTAL**
History & Physical				8–12%
Diagnostic studies				8–12%
Diagnosis				8–12%
Prognosis				8–12%
Managing patients				
Health maintenance				5–9%
Clinical intervention				18–22%
Clinical therapeutics				12–16%
Legal and ethical issues				4–8%
Applying basic concepts				8–12%
TOTAL	20–30%	55–65%	10–20%	100%

Source: USMLE.

dealing with the CCS portion of the USMLE 3. And, as noted earlier, the Primum® software package used in this part of the test will be sent to each USMLE 3 registrant beforehand. You must become thoroughly familiar with this software. At the time of writing this book, a good review of how to use this software was available on the NBME's Website at *www.nbme.org/new.version/prim.htm* under the menu tab "Primum software instruction review®." This is a young Web page, and changes are sure to be made over time.

Since you will be in the United States when you take this examination, it should not be difficult to get hands-on experience using a computer. Try going to the local library in the area where you are staying. Most libraries have computers available for public use, and you can usually get computer experience there with the assistance of library personnel. You should familiarize yourself with the following details of the computer and the CCS program:

1. The mouse. This is a gadget that moves the cursor or arrow on the computer screen. The mouse has a ball on its undersurface which moves the cursor when dragged along a flat surface. You

should drag the cursor to the spot that you choose and click on the front part of the mouse (left mouse button) to make that choice.

2. The keyboard. You should know where the "control," "page up," "page down," and other function keys are located. With computers, the same function can be performed by more than one maneuver on the keyboard or with the mouse. This knowledge can save you a lot of time during CBT and CCS.
3. Scrolling. You should be familiar with the strip on the right that is used to scroll up or down on the page.
4. The menu bar. The top of the computer screen has some words appearing horizontally. This is called the menu. For the CCS, the top row will read:

   File Clock Actions Windows Notepad Help

   You can perform a group of functions by going to each head (menu tab). To do so, take the cursor to that tab and press on the mouse button, which will show different functions under that heading in the form of a vertical column (drop-down menu). Drag the mouse, while pressing down the mouse button, to highlight the desired selection. Then release the mouse button. Some computers may require you to double click while on the highlighted area before you can make that choice. Practice on the CCS software and be fully aware of these functions before you go in to take the test. Study the explanations under the "Help" menu carefully.
5. The icon bar. The horizontal row below the menu bar contains various icons. In the CCS, different icons are used representing the history and physical exam, patient chart, order sheet, time, and patient location.

History and Physical Examination (H & P)

Once you press the icon for H & P, you will see the main heads titled "brief history," "comprehensive history," "interval/follow-up history," and "complete physical." Each main heading is preceded by a small square (☐). Each screen will display only the details of the item whose preceding square contains an X (☒). Clicking OK on the lower part of the screen will display the details of the item with an X in the square. As in real-life situations, getting the H & P will cost you some time. The computer will indicate the amount of time that will be added to your clock with acquisition of different pieces of data.

The interval history is the simulation of the situation in which a patient initially seen by you has a new complaint or change in condition.

Test/Therapy

Once you have made up your mind about the differential diagnosis, you may be ready to order tests and initiate therapy. By clicking on the appropriate icon, you will be able to order these tests as well as the initial therapy. You should write each new order on a new line. When you finish writing the orders, click on "confirm orders." You will then see screens on which you will have to specify the route, frequency, and so forth, for the previous orders. You should practice doing these maneuvers with the CCS software.

Order Sheet Request

You can click on "Help" to learn how to order tests and therapies; to check the results of order requests, and to cancel the orders.

Time

The area to the right of the time icon (in form of a clock) at the top of the screen displays the time. The time will change in the different ways as described below. You should be proficient with the following features before you take the exam.

- The clock simulates the time spent on various actions. As an example, when you are about to see the history on the screen, the computer will indicate that the clock will advance a specific number of minutes. Thus, although you are not taking the history yourself, it would have taken you this amount of time to obtain the information that the computer is going to give you. The same holds true for other parts of the H & P and for diagnostic tests. Thus, if you want to know the results of various tests, the computer will indicate how much time it will take to get the results for each test ordered. If you choose to see the results of a test or order a procedure, the clock will be advanced, and once advanced, it cannot be turned back. Your approach here should reflect how you would act in real-life situations. For example, if you are dealing with a patient with an acute problem and you happen to order a test whose result will not be in for 2 months, you should choose not to see those results as you cannot wait 2 months before initiating therapy.

- The clock keeps ticking in real time while you are reading the data on the screen. Therefore, you should practice reading this information quickly.
- The clock has a feature called "time advancing." In real-life situations, you would follow the results of tests ordered on your patients. You might also want to see a patient at a later date for follow-up. Or, you might want to see a patient after a specific period of time to see whether the therapy had taken effect or to look for any serious side effects of the therapy. The time advance feature lets you advance the clock for these purposes.
- Another clock feature is the "suspend time" function. Suppose you schedule a patient to be seen after, say, 3 months. In the interim you may receive lab or radiology results or the patient may call you with new complaints or questions. Based on this information, you may have to deal with a new situation. At other times, the information may not change the line of action. CCS simulates these situations. When you advance the time to simulate seeing a patient after a certain amount of time, the computer provides a simulation of the information you would receive in the intervening period. If the information demands a change of the line of management, you can then "suspend" the time clock and take action earlier than you had originally intended.
- You can schedule follow-up appointments on the computer using the calendar function. You should familiarize yourself with this feature.

Reviewing the Chart

The various features under this head are displayed in the various boxes (menu tabs) at the bottom of the screen. These tabs are displayed in the form of a horizontal strip which appears something like this:

		Order		Previous orders	
Order sheet	Progress notes	Lab reports	Imaging studies	Misc. tests	Vital signs

You can obtain different pieces of information by clicking on different areas, as follows:

- Order sheet: You can find information for placing, reviewing, and canceling orders here. The new orders can only be entered on the order sheet.
- Program notes: This tab displays old records if available. It also contains information regarding all the actions you have taken thus far.
- Lab results: This tab provides you with previous lab results.
- Imaging studies: These include ultrasound, nuclear medicine, x-ray, CAT scan, and MRI results.
- Misc. tests: This tab depicts the results of tests that do not require collecting specimens or visual imaging (e.g., ECG, spirometry, and psychometric testing results).
- Vital signs: This tab is self-explanatory.
- Previous orders: This tab informs you about all the clinical orders whose results have been seen. It also displays canceled orders.

None of these menu tabs can be used to solicit new information

Patient Location

This is a separate icon on the top of the screen. By clicking on it you can transfer the patient between the following locations as warranted: home, office, ward (hospital floor), ED, and ICU.

Case-end Instructions

At a preprogrammed stage, a box will appear stating that you have 5 real-time minutes before your case will be ended. During this time, you can delete or add orders or modify orders relevant to the latest condition of the patient. At the end of this time, you will be asked to enter the diagnosis before the case is closed. The appearance of the case-end instructions just means that the case has reached its programmed conclusion. It does not mean that you have done well or badly for this test item.

Exiting/Quitting the Case

You can finish the case before the case-end instructions in two different ways. One is by exiting the case. Pressing on the "File" tab at the top of screen and dragging the mouse to highlight the "Exit" can achieve this. By doing so, however, you will abruptly stop the case and not receive any credits that you might have gotten by continuing to manage the patient.

The other way to exit is to advance the clock. You will receive all the information about the change in patient's condition during this time. In this way, you will still have the opportunity to manage the patient over the simulated time axis.

PREPARING FOR THE EXAM

The USMLE 3 is an exam with its own unique flavor. Keep the following points in mind as you are preparing to take this test:

1. The test presumes that you have had some residency experience in the United States. The next chapters in this book should help you prepare better by giving you more information about the residency in the United States.
2. While it is very important to be knowledgeable about the subjects tested in the USMLE 1 and 2, there is a major difference between these tests and the USMLE 3. In the USMLE 1 and 2, you are given a scenario and expected to make the diagnosis. In the USMLE 3, the management of different situations is the main issue.
3. You should know the clear-cut answer to the main problems. As an example, you should know the best therapy for classic, run-of-the-mill, community-acquired pneumonia even though ten different antimicrobials might suffice to treat the condition.
4. Because of number 2 above, many examinees find it more useful to review material in ambulatory care or family practice books. This in no way negates the wealth of information in the big textbooks. You should read those books to develop a better understanding of the various disease entities.
5. Go with the obvious; do not go digging for "tricks" in these items.

The information bulletin for the USMLE 3 includes a useful list of topics according to different organ systems which you should use as a guide in preparing for the exam. The preceding information should help you fashion an effective study style while reading about these topics. The outline of topics that follows is intended to emphasize the importance of these areas; this should in no way take the place of reviewing the information provided in the USMLE booklet.

Eye:

- Red eye
- Ophthalmological signs of systemic diseases
- Awareness of macular degeneration as the most common cause of blindness among the elderly population in the United States
- Painful eye (e.g., glaucoma)

ENT (Ear, Nose, and Throat):

- Common ENT problems in children and adults (e.g., otitis media)
- Sore throat and its appropriate management

Central Nervous System:

- Aggressive management of stroke. In the United States today, a campaign is underway to replace the prevalent defeatist attitude toward stroke with a more aggressive approach similar to that used to treat myocardial infarction.
- Common degenerative diseases, including Parkinson's and Alzheimer's and awareness of their accompanying signs and symptoms. You should also be aware of various measures that can improve the quality of life for these patients.

Respiratory System:

- Sarcoidosis
- Home oxygen therapy: There is evidence to prove that home O_2 is useful in the treatment of patients with COPD. Medicare pays for O_2 for patients who meet certain criteria. These criteria are based on scientific evidence reviewed by the Health Care Financing Administration (HCFA).

    1. Patients must meet the following criteria to be eligible for home oxygen therapy:

        a. PaO_2 less than or equal to 55 mm Hg or pulse oximetry (SaO_2) less than or equal to 88 percent while awake, at rest, and breathing room air

        b. PaO_2 between 56 and 59 mm Hg or SaO_2 equal to 89 percent with evidence of any of the following:

i. Dependent edema suggesting congestive heart failure (CHF)
ii. P pulmonale on ECG (P wave more than 3 mm high in standard leads II, III, aVF)
iii. Hematocrit greater than 56 percent

2. Eligibility criteria for nocturnal oxygen are PaO_2 less than or equal to 55 mm Hg or SaO_2 less than or equal to 88 percent for a patient whose SaO_2 is better than 89 percent and PaO_2 is better than or equal to 56 mm Hg while awake. Other criteria include a sleeping PaO_2 that falls by more than 10 mm Hg or an SaO_2 that falls by more than 5 percent with signs or symptoms attributable to hypoxia, (e.g., impaired cognitive process, nocturnal restlessness, insomnia)
3. The criteria for O_2 only during exercise are PaO_2 less than or equal to 55 mm Hg or SaO_2 less than or equal to 88 percent during exercise. There should be additional evidence that the use of supplemental oxygen during exercise improves the hypoxemia demonstrated during exercise.

- Diagnosis and management of community- and hospital-acquired pneumonia based on the host characteristics
- Treatment of asthma based on its severity and including patient education issues
- Pulmonary embolism and various management issues, including diagnosis
- Sleep apnea syndrome; Its diagnosis and treatment, including nocturnal bilevel positive airway pressure (bipap).

Circulatory System

- Hypertension management in different situations: The Joint National Committee on Detection, Education, and the Treatment of High Blood Pressure periodically updates its treatment guidelines, which are well respected. You should be aware of the latest recommendations. At the time of writing of this book, JNC VI was the most recent; the guidelines can be found at Archives of Internal Medicine 1997;157:2413.
- Preventive cardiology: You should be aware of the management of modifiable risk factors for coronary artery disease (CAD).
- Management of a patient with chest pain, from diagnosis to appropriate management.

- Management of patients who are "skipping beats"; in other words, outpatient management of dysrrhythmias

Hematology

- Iron-deficiency amenia: The laboratory diagnosis, determination of its etiology, treatment, and indications for blood transfusion
- Diagnosis and management of vitamin B_{12} and folic acid deficiency and familiarity with all aspects of pernicious anemia
- Diagnosis and management of lymphoma and chronic lymphocytic leukemia (CLL) according to stage

Gastrointestinal System

- Barrett's esophagus: Its association with reflux, management, and follow-up.
- Diverticulitis, which is a common disease in the United States
- The best modality for diagnosing gallstones or cholecystitis
- Various criteria for the severity of pancreatitis; the best modality for the initial diagnosis or the diagnosis and management of various complications

Musculoskeletal System

- Indications for joint tap, and the findings in effusions of different etiologies
- Management of chronic back pain: Not every patient with back pain should have a CT scan or spinal x-ray. You should know the indications for more aggressive workup. If you have access to the Internet, you will find useful information at *www.ahcpr.gov*. This Web site contains various guidelines issued by the Agency for Health Care Policy and Research (AHCPR). Review the guidelines on acute low back problems in adults.
- Rotator cuff injuries

Renal Function

In the United States, many patients undergo chronic dialysis. Thanks to scientific advancements, these patients are living longer. You should be knowledgeable about basic aspects of management of patients on chronic dialysis, and be able to diagnose potential complications in a dialysis patient.

Reproductive System

- Pap smear: Its indications and interpretation
- Diagnosis of malignancies of various reproductive organs, and their management according to the stage
- Pelvic inflammatory disease
- Patient education regarding safe sexual practices
- Management of a testicular mass, including the correct diagnostic modality, and histology- and stage-appropriate treatment

Infectious Diseases

- AIDS and HIV-positive patients: The diagnosis, follow-up, and management of various complications; appropriate therapy for AIDS, including medications used to prevent opportunistic infections according to various stages of the disease
- Bacteria causing different infectious diseases; for cases where different bacteria may cause the same disease, you should know the most frequent cause.
- Diagnosis and treatment of sexually transmitted diseases; preventive measure and the education of patients
- Lyme disease
- Genitourinary tract infection, including cystitis and pyelonephritis; the choice of antibiotics and the duration of therapy in different situations

Trauma and Toxicology

- Management of a rape victim, including both physical and psychological aspects
- Common drug overdoses
- Toxic effects of nonmedicinal substances
- Toxicity of illicit drugs
- Priority-based management of trauma victims

Behavioral and Emotional Problems

- Common psychiatric disorders

- Anorexia nervosa and bulimia: the ability to diagnose from subtle signs
- Alcoholism and drug dependence: Diagnosis and the management
- Anxiety, mood and personality disorders: The emphasis is on the ability to diagnose on the basis of your interviews. You should also know the management of these disorders.
- Altered mental status: Diagnosis of delirium and its possible etiology
- Unconscious patient

Pregnancy and Childbirth

- Teen pregnancy, meaning pregnancy in an adolescent female: You should be aware of its psychosocial and economic coordinates.
- Abortion and its complications
- The progress of a normal pregnancy
- The common complications during pregnancy (e.g., placenta previa, abruptio placentae, eclampsia, pre-eclampsia)
- Management issues in high-risk pregnancy; Rh incompatibility
- Surveillance for suspected fetal abnormalities
- Normal delivery
- Normal puerperium and complications likely to occur during this period

Neonatology

- Congenital abnormalities: Their detection and management
- Apgar score
- Common problems in the perinatal period, including jaundice and infections, and their diagnosis during this period
- Problems of prematurity

Health Maintenance

This topic includes various activities that are explained later in this book.

Other Topics

- Abdominal pain
- Appropriate diagnostic tests for and management of a breast lump
- Diagnosis of physical abuse of elderly patients
- Problems common to an elderly population, such as urinary or bowel incontinence, frequent falls, polypharmacy, pressure ulcers, and so on
- Diagnosis on the basis of common signs and symptoms attributable to different systems (e.g., shortness of breath, cough, joint pain, chest pain, swelling of the feet, etc.)

Carefully study the list of topics provided in the information bulletin for the USMLE 3.

CHAPTER 9

Getting Into a Residency Program

Once you have met the criteria for ECFMG certification, you are ready to turn to the work of getting into a residency program. This is one of the most crucial steps in your endeavor to come to the United States. The residency is the first step in your career in the United States. The program you are admitted to will determine the type of fellowship or job you get after completion of the residency. It will also influence your family and personal life during the 3 years of your training. I cannot emphasize too strongly the importance of this step. Still, I have seen very few IMGs who give it more than a passing thought. There are several reasons for this oversight:

- IMGs know they are entering a market where the supply of potential candidates far exceeds the demand. So, they think that they are not in the position of being choosy.
- At the time they enter the United States, most IMGs feel that no sacrifice is too great to make in return for the chance to receive training in this country.
- Most of the literature available to IMGs lacks information about the pros and cons of various programs. The only way they learn hard realities of life as a resident in the United States is through first-hand experience. At that point, there is not a whole lot one can do.

Despite the adverse supply-and-demand scenario, every IMG who is admitted into a residency program in the United States has the choice of expressing a preference for one program over another. All that is lacking is an awareness of the key aspects to be considered in choosing the best program.

THE PROBLEM OF LOW SCORES

I have met many IMGs who are ECFMG certified but have not been able to get into a residency program because of their low USMLE scores. This can be a frustrating situation, especially for those IMGs who are already in the United States. It is also a sad waste of resources. The bitter remarks from this subset of people range from threats to filing a class-action lawsuit against ECFMG to decrying the USMLE for robbing people of their money by charging high exam fees. This book would be failing in its mission if I did not discuss this problem.

WHY ARE THE SCORES SO IMPORTANT?

The question asked by some IMGs is why their scores should matter so much when this does not seem to be the case for American medical graduates. Actually, scores do matter for U.S. graduates if they want to be accepted into a competitive residency program. However, they are more important for IMGs for the following reasons:

- Unlike the situation with U.S. graduates, most programs do not know anything about the medical school you graduated from. They do not know the scoring or evaluation system for the medical students in your country. They do not know what playing "college-level" football in Egypt means. In this scenario, the program director (PD) has to choose 100 candidates to interview out of the 2,000 applications he or she receives. What criteria can the PD use? Obviously, the ones that he or she is familiar or comfortable with. The USMLE score seems to be an easy choice.
- There is a feeling among many PDs that candidates with better USMLE scores have higher chances of passing the board exam, and board-pass percentage is one of the criteria for evaluating the standards of a residency program. This acts as a reinforcing factor for some PDs in the absence of any other criteria for evaluating most of the IMGs.

SHOULD THE SCORES MATTER AS LONG AS I AM ECFMG CERTIFIED?

If I were a PD, my answer might be, "I don't know. But can you provide any other criteria that I will feel more comfortable with?"

DOES A SCORE OF 75/75 MEAN THE END OF MY PROSPECTS FOR BECOMING A DOCTOR IN THE UNITED STATES?

No! If you have read the preceding paragraphs you will appreciate that the key to being accepted into a program is giving the evaluator some criteria that will impress him or her. Your score is obviously not going to do this, nor will your high ranking in high school. The first step toward developing a winning strategy is a ruthless reality check. Realize that:

1. With your score you probably do not have much chance of getting dozens of interview calls.
2. Your application is less likely to be noticed in a pile of applications. The Electronic Residency Application Service (ERAS) has made things more difficult in this regard. No longer can you attract attention with fancy stationary or an interesting format. In fact, some PDs who are very particular about scores do not even download applications with a score below the cutoff they have specified. The computer helps them in this initial screening process. So your application may not be looked at even if your performance in other fields has been stellar.

WHAT CAN I DO?

Your best chance is to select one or two programs and work relentlessly towards securing acceptance to them. Tips for improving your odds of being admitted into a program are listed in Table 9–1.

TABLE 9–1. Special Tips for Candidates with Low USMLE Scores

- ❑ Select one or two programs. Try to meet one of the people who have the biggest say in the resident selection process. Keep in mind that most people are afraid of commitment. Present yourself in a way that does not make these individuals feel they are obliged to accept you for a residency position. Use your meeting to find out if the decision makers take the USMLE scores as gospel. If so, look for another program.
- ❑ Do not sit in a basement and blindly start cranking out research papers, for that is where you may remain for the rest of your life. My personal opinion is that research is likely to prove helpful only in one of the conditions explained in Chapter One.
- ❑ Be visible. Once you have chosen a target program, work hard to present yourself in a positive light. You should be seen as honest, a good team player, courteous, hard working, and knowledgeable. By knowledgeable I do not mean that you should interrupt others in the middle of talking to distribute your own personal pearls.
- ❑ The bottom line is that you must ensure that you are seen as a complete human being rather than as just another entity stamped with a USMLE score. You can do this yourself by following the steps above or someone who is known to the decision maker can do this for you.

(continued on next page)

TABLE 9–1 Special Tips for Candidates with Low USMLE Scores (*continued*)

- ❑ When calling program coordinators, do not begin your conversation by asking, "Do you have a cutoff score?" If they do not, they may think about it after your call!
- ❑ Do not get hung up on your score. A low score may just mean that you are not a good exam taker. This generally has little to do with how good a doctor you will be.
- ❑ Look at yourself and the people around you. How many times have you or someone you know made up for one weakness by being very strong somewhere else? If a tennis player has an inherently weak backhand, he or she starts working on developing a killer forehand. That is the principle we have used so many times in our lives; why not now?

Getting into a residency program involves three steps, which will be considered in detail in the rest of this chapter:

1. The application process
2. Choosing among the residency programs
3. The interview process

Your application has only a few minutes to catch the evaluator's eye.

THE APPLICATION PROCESS

Let us imagine what it is like to be the PD or one of the subordinates who is responsible for deciding which applicants to interview for residency positions. This, by the way, is one of the many duties this person has to perform in his or her hospital. He or she takes time out from many other pressing issues and finally decides to sit down and dig through the piles of applications. He or she must decide which applicants are worthy of an interview call. Depending on how the particular program works, this person may either be the final authority or he or she may have to present a list of possible candidates to a panel of people. The evaluator has hundreds, possibly thousands, of applications to sift through and yours is one of them. You will probably have only a few minutes to make a sales pitch through your application. In these few minutes, you must convince this person to call you for an interview. The evaluator in all probability does not know the quality of the medical school from which you graduated, nor does he know how your cultural background will influence your ability to cope with the demands of a U.S. residency. There are so many questions that must be answered in a few minutes, and even in this era of sophisticated computer effects, your presentation is in the form of few simple pages printed from your ERAS application. Isn't this scary?

WHAT IS ERAS?

ERAS is an acronym that stands for the Electronic Residency Application Service. This service is run and managed by the Association of

American Medical Colleges (AAMC). For IMGs, ECFMG acts as a routing agency.

ERAS is a relatively new addition to the residency application process. Applicants are no longer required to send separate paper applications to the programs that use this service. Instead, they complete an application form on floppy disks, specifying the programs they want to apply to. The disks are sent to ERAS, which then directs the application to the specified programs for a charge that depends on the number of programs applied to.

You must apply for most residency programs through ERAS even if you receive an interview call through personal contacts.

As of 1999, ERAS will be used by most residency programs in:

Diagnostic radiology
Emergency medicine
Family practice
Internal medicine (preliminary and categorical)
Obstetrics and gynecology
Orthopedic surgery
Transitional year programs
Combined internal medicine–family practice
Combined internal medicine–emergency medicine

This list is likely to grow with time. Programs that do not appear on the list published at the time of your application require that the application be submitted the old-fashioned way.

HOW DOES ERAS WORK?

Applying through ERAS involves the following steps:

Step 1: Request the application materials from ECFMG. This will be in the form of floppy discs. Some of these discs (at the time of writing, this consists of three black floppy discs) contain software to be downloaded to your computer. Other discs (at this time, two white discs) are provided on which you will save your application information.
Step 2: Download this software onto a computer and type in the requested application information on the floppies provided. Decide which programs you want to apply to.
Step 3: Send the floppies back to ECFMG.
Step 4: Send any additional information later using a backup disc.

Once you have completed the residency application through ERAS, this information becomes available (through the computer) to the programs you have applied to. Upon receipt of your application, the PDs will make a decision about whether to call you for an interview. Beyond that, the process is almost the same as it was before ERAS, except that now you may receive interview calls by e-mail.

COMPUTERESE

If you do not have access to a computer that can run the ERAS program, you will need to make arrangements to use one that can.

ERAS has almost completely replaced the old-fashioned way of applying for a residency using a paper application. Having to "do it all" on the computer may scare some people. Following is a list of computer-related paraphernalia you will need to have before you can apply for residency through ERAS.

- To be able to use your computer for ERAS, the minimum requirements are: 486DX or higher PC-compatible computer capable of running Microsoft Windows 3.1 or higher, 8 MB RAM, 3.5-inch floppy disc drive, and a hard disc with 10 MB of file space. Your system should also be connected to a printer.
- Once you have access to such a computer, you can install the program for completing the application by following some easy commands.
- You do not need Internet access to complete the application. However, having such access will enable you to easily follow up on the status of your application. You should also have an e-mail address. That makes it easy for you to communicate with programs and vice versa. It is quite easy to set up an e-mail address, and various agencies and search engines offer free Web addresses. If you have access to the Internet, you can go to Web sites such as *www.hotmail.com* or *www.yahoo.com* to set up a free e-mail account. You can access this e-mail account from any computer that has Internet access.

GETTING THE APPLICATION MATERIALS

A form for requesting the ERAS application kit is available on line. You can print it by going to *www.ecfmg.org*. Depending on your mode of payment of the processing fee, you can send the completed form to these addresses:

- If you are enclosing a check or money order, mail it to: ECFMG ERAS Program, P.O. Box 820010, Philadelphia, PA 19182-0010, USA.
- If you are paying by credit card, fill in the credit card authorization and mail it to: ECFMG ERAS Program, P.O. Box 13467, Philadelphia, PA 19101-3467, USA, and fax the top of the form to 215-222-5641.

You can also request the ERAS kit by writing to:

ECFMG ERAS Program
P.O. Box 13467
Philadelphia, PA 19101-3467, USA

You will receive an instruction manual as a part of the kit. Look through the manual under the heading "Contents of SWS Kit." Be sure you have received everything as enumerated there. As a general rule, IMGs should receive the SWS program installation kit apart from the data diskettes. Some IMGs have gotten wrong diskettes. If you do not know what you are supposed to have, you can waste a lot of time troubleshooting.

ELIGIBILITY CRITERIA FOR APPLYING THROUGH ERAS

According to ECFMG, you can apply through ERAS as long as you have passed the USMLE Step 1 or have registered for the exam. However, you must have satisfied all the requirements for ECFMG certification before any program will show any genuine interest in you. Just being enrolled in ERAS is not enough.

FEES

You must pay a nonrefundable fee of $75 to obtain the application kit. At the time you submit the completed application, you will then have to pay an additional fee according to the number of programs you apply to. The fee computation is as follows:

- $60 for the first 10 programs applied to in *each* specialty. The word "each" is worth emphasizing here. For example, if you apply to three internal medicine programs, three family practice programs, and four radiology programs, the total number of programs is only 10, but you will have to pay $180 because you have to pay at the rate of $60 for the first ten programs in each of these three specialties.

- $6 each for the next 10 programs (programs 11 to 20) in each specialty. Again, if you apply to 15 programs in internal medicine, you will pay $60 for the first 10 and $5 × 6 = $30 for the next five programs, for a total of $90.
- $12 each for the next 10 programs (programs 21 to 30) in each specialty.
- $30 each for programs 31 and up in each specialty.

Let us suppose you want to apply to 50 programs in internal medicine. Your calculation would be as follows:

$60 for the first ten programs
$60 for programs 11 to 20
$120 for programs 21 to 30
$600 for programs 31 to 50 (at the rate of $30 each)
Total: $840

Boy, that hurts! Especially when you realize that most IMGs apply to at least 50 programs to maximize their chances of getting into a program.

INSTALLATION

Once you have received the kit, you will need to install it on the computer. The instruction manual gives simple step-by-step instructions for installing the software. The problem I foresee for many IMGs is lack of access to a computer. Try to use a computer at school, in the library, or at a friend's place. One problem with computers available for public use is that often these computers do not allow users to install additional software on to the machine. You might try talking to the individual in charge and explaining that this program is academic software and it does not use up much of the hard disc space.

If possible, keep the software loaded on the computer; you may need more than one session to complete the application and may also want to update it later. If you have problems convincing the owner of the computer to keep the software on the hard drive, offer to de-install it after use. You can either try to finish the application in one sitting or reinstall it from the discs as often as necessary.

USING THE ERAS PROGRAM

Once you have gone through the simple steps of installing the software, you are ready to use it. First, put in the student's data disc. This will bring up the menu of options available on the disc. The menu will read something like this:

Save work	Help
Work on CAF	Check application completeness
USMLE score	Print application
Get program information	Print CV
Select programs	Print invoice
Personal statement	Program selection report
Letters of recommendation	Application complete certification
Assign documents	Exit

You can carry out the function performed by each option by moving your cursor to that item and clicking there. The various functions are described below.

1. Save Work

Clicking on this option saves all your work onto the floppy disc. You should save your work at the end of each session. But *do not* certify it. Once you have certified the disc, you will not be allowed to make further changes to the information on the same disc.

2. Work on CAF

CAF stands for complete application form. Once you click on this option, you will see a menu like the following:

Previous resid.	Work exper.	Volunteer exper.	Research	Publications	Medical licensure	Examinations
General 1	General 2	General 3	General 4	Undergraduate educ.	Graduate educ.	Medical educ.

Previous Residency. When you click on this category, you will pull up boxes in which to write about all the training you received after medical school.

Work Experience. Enumerate any jobs held as a medical professional apart from those that involved training.

Volunteer Experience. This category should include any work done without any direct financial remuneration. This could include activities such as taking part in providing free health checkups for the poor. If you will be living in the United States for a while before sending in this application, you can volunteer for various organizations working, for example, with the mentally challenged, cancer patients, and so on.

Research. This part of the application allows you to list any research you have carried out. The format requires you to enter the name of the organization you worked with and the time period during which you did that research. Thus, if you did research while in medical school, you should put down your school's name under the heading for organization. This category can be problematic if you did research during a period when you were not associated with any organization. In such cases, you may write the name of a co-researcher's organization.

Publications. Here you should enumerate all of your publications. You should also list any articles you have submitted for possible publication at the time of the application.

Medical Licensure. Specify any license to practice medicine you may have received in your country.

Examinations. This category simply asks you about your USMLE exam history.

General 1, 2, and 3. This category asks for your personal information. Be sure you have an e-mail address to include here.

General 4. Here you can summarize your hobbies and interests. Do not try to tailor your hobbies to those you think might be attractive to the PD. There is always a chance that others will have the same hobbies as you. If you are wondering whether your hobbies are too offbeat, consider this: you at least have a shot at getting the other person intrigued about your "weirdness"—and that is not a bad thing to start with. In the same section, there is a box for enumerating "other accomplishments"; this is the place where you can fit in all the things you think are important but for which no space is set aside in the form.

Undergraduate Education, Graduate Education. Just enumerate the basic information in these categories.

Medical Education. Apart from simple information, you are also allowed to mention all the honors and awards you received in medical school. The space here is limited, so you may have to prioritize to get in what you think is most important.

3. USMLE Score

In this column, just indicate that you want the examination authorities to send the exam results to the concerned programs. This is done for a fee that is added to the amount you pay for the application process.

4. Get Program Information

Here you can obtain detailed information about various programs offering residency positions. The box asks you to select three pieces of information: type of program, state where the program is located, and discipline.

a. Type of program: There are four types of programs, as follows:

- Categorical (C): These are programs in which, once you have been selected, you can continue up to the completion of training required for specialty certification. This is the type of program preferred by most IMGs because, once in, they have the security of being able to complete their training.
- Preliminary (P): These programs provide 1 or 2 years of prerequisite training for entry into advanced positions in the specialty programs that require 1 or more years of broad clinical training in internal medicine. Such specialties include anesthesiology, neurology, emergency medicine, OB/GYN, pediatrics, psychiatry, and radiology. Some of the programs offering residency in these specialties also offer preliminary positions. If you are

planning to enter one of these specialties, you must secure a preliminary as well as an advanced position.

Note: IMGs sometimes accept preliminary positions without having an advanced position offer in hand. They do this to "get a foot in the door." While for some IMGs this could easily end up as a dead-end job, in very desperate situations, it may not be a bad move.

- Advanced position (S): These are the positions in the programs that begin after the completion of 1 or more years of preliminary training. Let us say you begin your neurology residency application process in August of 2001. You would apply for the P position in medicine which starts in July 2002 and the advanced position in neurology which starts in 2003 at the same time—August 2001.
- Physician (R) positions: These are the positions offered to physicians who have had prior graduate medical education in the United States. I will not elaborate further as readers are not likely to belong to this group.

b. The next step is choosing the state where the program of interest to you is located. The diskette gives you the standard postal code abbreviations for various U.S. states, not their complete names. For example, Illinois is IL and Minnesota is MN. This can be confusing to IMGs. Following is a list of the states and their abbreviations.

Alabama	AL	Hawaii	HI
Alaska	AK	Idaho	ID
Arizona	AZ	Illinois	IL
Arkansas	AR	Indiana	IN
California	CA	Iowa	IA
Colorado	CO	Kansas	KS
Connecticut	CT	Kentucky	KY
Delaware	DE	Louisiana	LA
District of Columbia	DC	Maine	ME
Florida	FL	Maryland	MD
Georgia	GA	Massachusets	MA

Michigan	MI	Oregon	OR
Minnesota	MN	Pennsylvania	PA
Mississippi	MS	Rhode Island	RI
Missouri	MO	South Carolina	SC
Montana	MT	South Dakota	SD
Nebraska	NE	Tennessee	TN
Nevada	NV	Texas	TX
New Hampshire	NH	Utah	UT
New Jersey	NJ	Vermont	VT
New Mexico	NM	Virginia	VA
New York	NY	Washington	WA
North Carolina	NC	West Virginia	WV
North Dakota	ND	Wisconsin	WI
Ohio	OH	Wyoming	WY
Oklahoma	OK		

c. The last step is to choose the discipline, for example, internal medicine, family practice, and so on.

d. Once you have done that, click on the button for "program info." You will receive the information about the program selected. This information is designed to help you make an informed decision about the programs you apply to.

5. Select Programs

This option lets you choose the programs you want to apply to.

6. Personal Statement

The personal statement, as its name implies, is a statement about you. In this section, you are asked to type in about a page worth of information about yourself. Many IMGs are very uncomfortable writing this statement. For one thing, many of us are brought up with the advice that bragging about ourselves is a bad thing, and saying only good things about yourself on a piece of paper sounds a lot like bragging. This is more so if you have never had to produce such a document to this point in your career. A personal statement should give at least the following information about you:

Your personal statement should have your *personal flavor.*

- ❑ Your academic and nonacademic achievements. This should not be a rehash of your CV. You have already included that document in the application kit.
- ❑ Why you are in the field of medicine and why you want to train in the field to which you are applying.
- ❑ What your plans are after you complete the training for which you are applying.

These areas do not need to be discussed under different headings in your statement, but instead can be interwoven together. Try to give the highlights of your achievements that are likely to work toward the same goal; that is, making you look like a better candidate for the job.

As a part of the personal statement, you should also write about what drove you to enter the field of medicine. Write anything you want except "my dad wanted me to". What is there about the specialty to which you are drawn that you like the most? Do some soul searching and come up with your own personal reasons.

You are coming to the United States with the obvious plan of obtaining good training. You should be able to state in concise form what you want to do after you complete this training. Tell your reader about your vision. Focus on where you would like to be in 5 or 10 years.

Do's and Don'ts of the Personal Statement

Don't . . .

- ❑ . . . make it look like your autobiography. It should be one page long. If your statement is longer than that, read it over and trim it down.
- ❑ . . . try to make it the exact replica of the statement of a friend who got into Stanford last year. Your personal statement has to be supported by data such as your age, experience, and the other things listed on your CV. Anyone who becomes a doctor has achieved a lot in his or her career. It is simply a question of focusing in on the good things. Different programs and even different persons in the same program may have different definitions of "good". So talk about the highlights of your career. Beyond that, it comes down to whether or not you "click" with the people reading your application. Let your personal statement have a flavor that is unique to your own self. In my experience, the problem is not having little to write but rather the inability to put it down on paper in an easily readable form. Remember that you have only a few minutes to make your sales pitch.

- ❑ . . . exaggerate about any of your accomplishments, thinking that people in the United States may not know the facts. First, the communication systems of today have made this world a very small place. Second, the person reading your statement may be from your own country.

Do . . .

- ❑ . . . put a lot of effort in writing your statement. Every line you write must imply that you are the best person for the job.
- ❑ . . . write different personal statements if you are applying for different specialties.

Computerese for Personal Statement. This section of the ERAS diskette allows you to write only in simple text or as an ASCII file. You can use only the Times New Roman or Courier New fonts. You may write your statement separately as text and then paste it into this section, or you can write here directly. This section does allow you to write more than one personal statement so that you can send different statements to different programs.

7. Letters of Recommendation

You are allowed to send a maximum of four letters of recommendation. The importance of these letters cannot be overemphasized. In the United States, opportunities for one's career advancement are often based at least partly on recommendations. This may be a new idea for IMGs from some parts of the world, where one's academic record alone can take one anywhere. Having come from India, I saw many of my friends who went to their professors to request letters of recommendation. Very often these professors do not know what to write that would be most helpful to their students in the United States. Another thing worth mentioning is that very often the person reading your letter will not know the person who wrote your letter of recommendation. Please request your letter writer to state his or her field of expertise in the opening lines of the letter. If your letter writer is known for particular achievements in his or her field of expertise these should also be listed as they give more credibility to this person's words. If you do not ensure inclusion of this information, those reading your letter may not recognize the reputation of your letter writer even if he or she has published hundreds of papers in respected journals.

The recommendation letter must contain all the essential parts to be effective.

Essential Parts of a Recommendation Letter. Obviously, this should be a truthful account of what the letter writer thinks about you. Following is the suggested format:

1. The letter should begin with a salutation such as "Dear doctor," or "To whom it may concern." ERAS does not allow you to send letters addressed to individual PDs by name.
2. The writer should then introduce himself or herself preferably giving a small account of his or her own accomplishments. Next, the letter writer should proceed by stating how long and in what capacity he or she has known you.
3. The letter writer should touch on the following areas:
   a. Your academic achievements.
   b. Your personal attributes such as professionalism, dependability, compassion, and so forth.
   c. Your fund of knowledge and how you apply it to actual patient care.
   d. Any research activities you have carried out; your communication skills and command of English.
   e. Anything you have done that was beyond the call of duty. This could be in the form of community work, management position, or anything of that sort.
   f. Anything else of a positive nature that the letter writer thinks is unique to you.
4. At the end, the letter writer should wholeheartedly recommend you as a candidate and should give his or her contact information (phone number or e-mail address) with an offer to discuss your qualifications in more detail. A letter stating that your performance was "satisfactory" or "okay" is pretty much taken as a negative recommendation.

Computerese for Letter of Recommendation. Clicking on the button for "letters of recommendation" enables you to type in the name and position of your recommenders one by one, up to the maximum of four. Then go to the "file" tab at the top left corner of your computer screen. By clicking on "print" from this menu, you can choose the specific recommendation letter cover sheets to print. The sheet for each separate letter of recommendation will contain the name of that letter writer. These sheets have an identifying bar code that connects them to your application. You would then send the appropriate sheet to each letter writer; he or she would send the actual letter of recommendation to ECFMG along with this cover sheet. Alternately, you would get the letters from your writers and send them along with your application kit. This latter approach assures timely arrival of all of your application materials at the same time.

Who Should Write Your Recommendation Letter? The letter writer must be a person who has observed you working as a medical student or postgraduate. It should preferably be a person from the specialty to which you are going to apply. An exception can be made if you are applying for a residency in medicine but your surgery teacher is world-renowned for his or her pioneering work in, say, hernia repair. It is always better if your letter writer is well respected in his or her academic field. As noted earlier, if this is the case, be sure the letter writer mentions his or her accomplishments at the start of the letter.

If possible, you should try to get one or more letters from doctors in the U.S. You can accomplish this by working with a United States doctor as an observer, researcher, or in another capacity. PDs tend to feel more secure giving credence to letters written by people who are working in the United States.

8. Assign Documents

This part of the diskette lets you assign different documents to different programs. Only the documents assigned to a particular program will be sent to that program. There are two important considerations here. The first concerns which programs you want to send your USMLE scores to. I recommend that IMGs assign these scores to each program. The second concerns your personal statement; this applies if you are applying to more than one specialty and have written a separate letter for each. *Make sure* that the radiology PD does not receive a personal statement from you saying, "I have dreamed of becoming an internist ever since I got out of diapers". (Pun intended.)

9. Help

This option includes different topics to help you fill out the application form and work through the program.

10. Check Application Completeness

This option checks your application for completeness and lets you know if you left out any requested information.

11. Print Application

This option enables you to print your application for your records.

12. Print CV

This option prints out the CV that the computer has created on the basis of information that you have entered.

13. Print Invoice

This option will print the invoice and tell you the amount (in U.S. dollars) that you need to send along with the diskette. The fee will be computed on the basis of the number of programs you are applying to.

14. Program Selection Report

This option gives you the list of programs that you choose.

15. Application Complete Certification

Certification should be done just prior to sending the diskette to ECFMG. Remember, once you have certified your application you cannot change any information on the diskette. At the time you certify the disc, it will prompt you to make a backup copy. The backup copy can be used to submit any changes in your application. ECFMG sends you one extra disc to use for this backup. If you need to send a second update, you can use a regular 3.5-inch floppy disc to create the backup.

16. Exit

This option is clicked whenever you want to exit after working on the diskette.

SENDING THE APPLICATION

Once you have completed the application, you will need to send it to ERAS at one of the following addresses:

1. If you are sending the disks and documents without a check or money order, you can send them to:

   ERAS Program
   P.O. Box 13467
   Philadelphia, PA 19101-3467 USA

2. If you *enclose a check or money order* with your disc, send the packet to:

   ERAS Diskettes at PNC
   P.O. Box 820010
   Philadelphia, PA 19182-0010 USA

3. For *courier delivery*, you can use the following address:

   ERAS Program
   3624 Market Street
   Philadelphia, PA 19104 USA

Key Issues Raised by the Introduction of ERAS

- ERAS necessitates access to a computer and the ability to use this software well. This could be a problem for some IMGs.
- Under ERAS, you will be charged according to the number of probrams to which you apply. This could mount up to a large sum. As a general rule, IMGs have to apply to more programs than U.S. medical graduates.
- ECFMG has provided an e-mail address that IMGs can use to seek help in case of a problem. In my personal experience with this feature, I either did not get a response to my query or the answer was in the form of a default response that did not really address the issue. I hope the usefulness of this new feature improves with time.
- Certain sections of ERAS place a cap on the number of characters that can be typed in by the applicant. This system also takes away the ability to use a distinct stationary or some other eye-catching feature.

CHOOSING AMONG THE PROGRAMS

DECIDING WHERE TO APPLY

Once you have decided which specialty you want to apply to, you have to choose from the programs offering that training. It is more important than ever before to be both thorough and discrete in your choice in view of the fee structure for ERAS. As previously noted, your application fee is now directly proportional to the number of programs to which you apply. Following are the main resources that describe the residency training programs available in the United States for different specialties.

- **ERAS Diskette**
  If you are applying to one of the programs that use ERAS, you will receive a full list of all of the residency programs available. It will even enumerate the programs, in the specialty of your choice, that are not using ERAS (those programs are set off by a gray background).
- **"Green Book"**
  This is a graduate medical education directory published by the American Medical Association (AMA). This book provides a detailed list of programs available all over the country.
- **FREIDA On-line**
  This is a Web site maintained by the AMA providing on-line information about all the programs. Apart from this information, you can also see statistics about the workforce in your chosen specialty. I found this to be a valuable tool. You can access it by going to *www.ama-assn.org*.
- **NRMP Book**
  Once you enroll with the National Residency Matching Program (NRMP), you will receive the latest information in the form of a listing of programs in different specialties. The problem is that you get this information around October, at a time when you should have already applied. Another point worth mentioning is that with NRMP going online for most of its operations, you may not receive enough information in hard-copy form from them.
- **Your Friends**
  This is an important resource. These are the friends who ask you to apply to the programs they are already in and are ready to follow up on your application with their PDs or the secretaries.

X, Y, Z OF THE PROGRAMS

You will find that the programs are divided into types X, Y, and Z. An X program means it is owned and operated by a university/LCME-accredited medical school. These are also called "university programs". Such programs are typically very well respected and are considered to be academically strong. This is helpful if you are planning to seek a fellowship or want to enter an academic field later. In addition, these programs are more likely to have big-name professors who can help further your career. On the downside, university programs are large programs. It is easy to become lost in those huge programs. As a general rule, university program residents typically staff busy hospitals.

A Y program is one that has an institutional agreement with an LCME-accredited medical school.

A Z program is one that has some department association but no institutional agreement with an LCME-accredited medical school. These programs are typically based in small hospitals that may not be very strong academically. It may be tougher to get a fellowship if you do your residency at such an institution. On the other hand, you may have a better relationship with your teachers. These hospitals may also provide better working conditions. Table 9–2 spells out several things you should consider before choosing the programs to which you will apply.

TABLE 9–2. Considerations in Deciding Where to Apply for a Residency

1. *What are your chances?*
   a. First of all, measure how tolerant the program is to IMGs. This is the most important consideration. If you are applying to a program that has never seen a foreign medical graduate and has no tearing urgency to see one, you may be wasting an application. Here are a few indicators of IMG tolerance:
      - The program has a history of accepting IMGs for training.
      - Programs in the larger cities are more likely to be tolerant of IMGs. Examples are most East Coast cities including New York; cities such as Detroit, St. Louis, and Chicago in the Midwest; and some places in the south such as Houston and Atlanta. West Coast programs have generally tried to deter IMGs. Of course, this list is not all-inclusive and I am giving you broad generalizations here. Sometimes you will find a single institution in an otherwise IMG-intolerant state or city that will respect and welcome IMGs.
      - Hospitals with a clientele from your same ethnic group may view you as an attractive candidate.

   b. The big-name university programs such as Stanford and Yale are harder to get into. This is true for all IMGs, but more so for those who are fresh from their country unless they can show some stellar achievements. You may be able to make inroads into such institutions if you are ready to spend an extra year or two in research.

(*continued*)

TABLE 9–2 Considerations in Deciding Where to Apply for a Residency (*continued*)

c. If you have carried out special research or have training in a particular field, try to apply to an institution that has a special interest in the same field.

2. *Where is it located?* The United States is a huge country. On any given day the temperature may register 75° F and −20° F at the same time in different parts of this country. Some regions of the country are covered with snow for most of the winter; others are known for very hot summers. Some regions have frequent tornadoes while others are more likely to have an earthquake. One area of a city may have a high crime rate while another area of the same city has one of the best school systems. You also should consider how tolerant a particular city is of foreigners. Some of these points may sound frivolous before you come to the United States. However, consider that once you are accepted into a residency program, you will need to cope with these day-to-day aspects of life in a foreign country. By learning from the experience of other IMGs, you can live life on your own terms and also improve the experience of being in the United States for your spouse and children.
3. *What type of program is it?* The program selection should be made according to your future plans. Consider the following:
   a. If you want to apply for a fellowship after residency, you should try to be accepted into a program with its own fellowship program. You always have a better chance of securing a fellowship in the program where you do your residency. If possible, you should join a program that has a good reputation for the specialty you want to train in later.
   b. Delve into the history of the program regarding if and to what extent they help their residents in furthering their careers.
   c. If you plan to begin practicing in the United States after completing your residency and you are eligible to do that, it may be fine to work in a small community hospital where you may be able to establish your professional credentials and gain clout over the years of your residency.

NATIONAL RESIDENCY MATCHING PROGRAM

Enrollment in the National Residency Matching Program (NRMP) is an almost indispensable part of the hunt for a residency. The steps in the NRMP are as follows:

1. Candidates enroll with the NRMP.
2. Most of the residency programs offering residency positions enroll with the NRMP. Some programs may offer their residency positions without going through the NRMP. Others may offer some of their positions without going through the NRMP and the rest of them through it.
3. Candidates as well as the programs run the interview process on their own. After this, the candidates rank the programs that they have interviewed for according to preference. The

programs do the same, and both parties independently send their ranking lists to the NRMP.

4. The NRMP matches the programs and candidates in a way that respects both parties' choices.

Enrolling with the NRMP

Enrollment in the NRMP opens approximately in June of the year prior to the start of training. For example, enrollment for programs starting in July of 2004 will begin around June 2003. You can enroll by going to the NRMP Web site at *http://eraspo5.aamc.org/nrmp* or by calling 202-828-0566 from 9 A.M. to 5 P.M., Eastern Standard Time, Monday through Friday. You can also communicate by writing to:

NRMP
2501, M Street, NW, Suite 1
Washington DC 20037 USA

Eligibility

You must have satisfied all the prerequisites for entry into residency in the United States before the NRMP will consider putting you in the matching pool. Nevertheless, you can enroll with the NRMP even if some steps are pending. Keep in mind that you will be considered for the match only if the NRMP receives information directly from ECFMG that you have passed all of the steps successfully. This information must reach the NRMP before the deadline for submission of the rank list. I will repeat that this information *must come* from ECFMG directly.

The Rank List

The NRMP does not play any part in securing interview calls. After you have interviewed at different places, you should submit your rank list, which includes programs in the descending order of your preference. You should list only those programs with whom you interviewed. Also, make sure that the residency programs you interviewed with are participating in the matching program. Some important guidelines are as follows:

1. If you are submitting the rank order list through the Internet, you do not have to wait until the last moment to submit it. The Internet allows you to modify the list as many times as you want before the deadline fixed by the NRMP.
2. You should prepare the rank list exactly in the order of your own preference. You should consider the factors enumerated later in this chapter in the section on "The Interview Process." It is a common misconception among applicants that they should rank high the programs they think will rank *them* high, even if they would prefer to put these at the bottom. This approach is erroneously thought to ensure a match. Let us suppose you put a program at number seven and the program puts you at number one and someone else puts the same program at number one. If you do not match with any one out of the top six of your choices, you will still match with that program ahead of this other person in the matching pool. The best advice is to make the list on the basis of where you would like to train, irrespective of anyone's assurances or dissuasion.
3. You can rank 15 programs for no extra charge. Beyond this, you have to pay $30 for each extra program matched. If you are one of the few lucky IMGs who has more than 15 interviews, but you want to rank only 15 programs, you may have to consider various factors such as competitiveness of the programs or the chosen specialty. Also, make sure that you only list the programs that you are ready to join. This may seem a bit comical to IMGs at this initial stage of their careers. But I have heard some unhappy residents say, "I would have preferred to wait 10 years rather than join this program".
4. The NRMP states that it prefers to accept the rank list almost exclusively through the Internet. If you do not have access to the Internet, you can call the NRMP at 202-828-0566 to make alternative arrangements. This near-total computerization of the residency matching process prompted one of my friends to say, "This seems to be a part of the bigger conspiracy [by the computer giants] to getting computers into the smaller countries of the world".

Match Results

The NRMP fixes a time on a particular day when candidates will be able to find out whether or not they matched. This can be done by logging onto the NRMP Web site or by calling the NRMP at 202-828-0566.

You will need your NRMP code and personal identification number (PIN) (which you will be given at the time of enrollment) to access the results on the Web or by phone. This system of making match results available immediately by electronic means has had the benefit of placing IMGs on a par with United States medical graduates. In years past, when applicants had to depend on the results coming by mail, IMGs often received their results days later with no chance in the postmatch scramble. A day or two later, at a time decided by the NRMP, the matched candidates find out *where* they matched.

Postmatch Scramble

This is the name for the process in which unmatched candidates try to get into one of the unfilled positions. Traditionally, about 24 hours after the match results are posted, a list of the programs that did not fill all their positions, and hence may be looking for candidates, becomes available. This information is critical to the applicants who do not match and, once again, it will be available to the registered candidates, only. Armed with this information, the candidates who did not match try to grab one of the unfilled seats.

The postmatch period can be a very stressful time, as candidates have a very limited time in which to act. A few helpful points are noted below:

- ❑ Be realistic. If you find a vacant spot in one of the institutions that you initially thought you had no chance of getting into, your chances of being accepted at this stage are probably still the same postmatch. You should not put your efforts into calling such programs first.
- ❑ Instead, if one of the places where you interviewed has a spot, try there first.
- ❑ Scout around for the places where you may know someone who can expedite your connection with the decision-making authorities. Remember that it is a very stressful and frustrating time for the institutions with unmatched spots, too.

DIAL-A-RESIDENCY

I am coining my own phrase to describe the phenomenon whereby IMGs sign a contract for a residency without coming to the United States for interviews. In most cases this is done by interviewing with the PD over the phone. This happens in situations where either the candidate has an international reputation or he or she knows an influential person in the United States who recommends him or her wholeheartedly. This phenomenon is becoming less and less common as residency spots in United States hospitals are shrinking. But it continues to occur in certain cases. There are pros and cons to signing the contract on the basis of a telephone interview. An advantage is that you do not have to go through the hassle of the interview process and you know you have a secure spot in a residency program. The disadvantage is that you might have been able to get a better deal if you had shopped around.

SIGNING PREMATCH

Sometimes during the interview process, residency programs may express interest in signing a contract with a candidate without having to go through the NRMP process. This happens in situations where PDs feel that the candidate is the type of person they would be happy to have but are not sure they will secure through the match.

This is a flattering position to be in. It also assures the IMG of a residency spot. It means no more expensive travel for interviews. The IMG can go back home and start preparing for the residency. However, if you find yourself in this position, I would suggest you request some time to think over the offer. If this is exactly the type of program you dreamed of getting into, there is no point in holding out just to see where else you might match. If not, try to think about your chances of getting into other programs that are more attractive to you.

Signing the residency contract "out of match" should be a well-thought-out and not an impulsive decision.

This may be a difficult situation because the surety of getting into *some* residency is the priority for most IMGs. The decision about whether or not to sign a contract "out of match" will probably always be taken by individuals on the basis of their own level of comfort with risk-taking, which in turn depends on a multitude of factors.

A few tips that may come in handy if you find yourself in the position of being offered an out-of-match contract follow.

- If you would rather go through the match, say so. Do not try to hedge your bets by leading on the PDs. There is a common feeling among IMGs that if a candidate refuses to sign out of match for a program, that program will not rank the candidate in the NRMP list. This idea may have been passed along from generation to generation of IMGs coming to the United States, or it may be prompted by subtle cues sent by offering programs that really want to sign up a particular candidate. I think PDs who know how to use the NRMP to their advantage always rank the most desirable interviewees at the top, even if they feel they may never get them. If you are the type of candidate they definitely want, they will rank you. Thus, if you think you would much rather do your residency somewhere else, do not let anyone psych you into signing where you do not want to. As long as you do not act disrespectfully or egotistically, you are unlikely to kill your chances with the offering program through the match. The one exception to all that I have said here is the program that has a history of signing nearly all its contracts prematch. In this case, the program may be willing to offer the position to next desirable candidate. Once again, it will be up to you to decide what risks you are willing to take.
- If you need more time before making your final decision, say so. Ask for additional time in which to think the offer over. PDs should understand that everyone deserves some time to make a decision as important as this one.

If you do decide to sign a contract prematch, *do not forget to withdraw your name from the NRMP pool*. If you do not, and you do get matched with another program, per NRMP rules, you are obliged to accept the residency with the latter program.

THE INTERVIEW PROCESS

Once you have applied to the residency programs, you should begin receiving interview calls. The interview process can be divided into four steps as shown in Table 9–3.

GETTING THE INTERVIEW CALLS

You should have applied to various residency programs based on the criteria enumerated earlier in this chapter. Oftentimes getting enough

TABLE 9–3. Steps in the Interview Process
1. Getting the interview calls
2. Scheduling the interviews
3. Getting through the interviews
4. Following up afterward

calls for interviews is the main concern of IMGs. Some IMGs may not be called for interviews despite having fulfilled all the requirements for starting a residency in the United States. Based on my research, the following suggestions can help better your chances of receiving sufficient interview calls.

Personal contacts are a very useful resource when trying to secure interview calls. Tap them.

1. Carefully choose the programs you apply to. Go through the checklist described earlier in Table 9–2 to get an idea about your chances of being accepted into those programs.
2. Try tracking down any of your friends or acquaintances who are physicians in the United States. Some of these people might help you secure an interview call by talking with their PDs or some other equally powerful person. Sometimes it is amazing how much difference a simple word from a helpful acquaintance can make. This is an amazing but quite understandable phenomenon. From a PD's perspective, you are otherwise just another piece of paper in the huge pile of applications. Once someone he or she knows says something about you, however, you suddenly become a person the PD can visualize. Call as many people as you know and send them a hard copy of your application materials. You should also have applied to these programs through ERAS.

   Note: One problem you may have during this process is not knowing how to contact your acquaintences. Most of these people initially move to one location in the United States, then obtain a residency somewhere else, and later move yet again to do a fellowship or start a practice. The following tips can help you trace your contacts in the United States.

- If you are in touch with other friends in the United States, ask them if they know the whereabouts of your common friends in the medical profession there.
- To locate the whereabouts of your physician friends, you can also try consulting the *Directory of Physicians in the United States* published by the AMA or going to the association's Web page at *www.ama-assn.org*.
- If you have access to Internet, you can search for persons by name and city in the United States. You may be able to find their phone numbers or e-mail addresses.
- If you know the exact place where the person you are looking for lives, try calling directory assistance for help. Dial the telephone area code for that place followed by 555-1212. This will connect you to directory assistance, which can check for a telephone listing for that person by his or her last name.

3. The steps involved in coming to the United States keep many IMGs from working as doctors for a while as they prepare to take the exams or apply to residency programs. Unfortunately, this period is sometimes looked at as a "break" in your career by PDs. You can avoid this type of gap by doing research or performing other medically related work, as mentioned in Chapter 1.
4. If you can, try to follow up with different programs after submitting your application. You can call them on the phone to ask if they have received your application. Some programs deem such follow up an expression of special interest in their program. Better yet, you can follow up by writing an e-mail to the various programs. This may have the advantage of helping to present you as a computer-savvy person.

SCHEDULING THE INTERVIEWS

Once you have received the interview calls, the next important step involves clever scheduling of the interviews. Keep the following points in mind:

- Try to schedule the dates and times for different interviews so that you do not have to travel back and forth to the same area time and again. If you receive an interview call from a program in one city and you have applied to other programs in that area, call these programs to see if they are planning to grant you an interview. Explain that you are asking because you will be in the area to interview someplace else. Most of the people you speak with should understand this situation, and these calls may save you extra trips.
- It can be very expensive to telephone from outside the United States. Try to schedule interview dates by e-mail as much as possible. Another option is to ask a friend in the United States to make these calls for you.
- If you have never interviewed in the United States and have several interviews lined up, the first interview you schedule should be at the program you are least interested in joining. This will act as your "warm-up" interview.
- If you are traveling from your country exclusively for the interviews and are looking for a prematch sign-up, try to interview around October. The reason for this is that programs offering prematch sign-ups like to secure residents during the early part of the interview season.
- If you are coming to the United States from your country to interview, make your travel plans while in your own country. Look into discounts on interstate travel in the United States. It is easier to do that at the time when you are buying your ticket for international travel. Moreover there are often bargains available to tourists visiting the United States. Your agent should be able to find these for you. Look also at the possibility of making travel arrangements through the internet.

DURING THE INTERVIEW PERIOD

Keeping in Touch

It is important to keep in touch with the folks back home as well as with friends in the United States while you are traveling for interviews. It can be outrageously expensive to make interstate or overseas calls from pay phones. Buy a phone card instead. These cards are sold by the number of minutes. You can usually purchase these at gas stations and convenience stores. Ask your acquaintances in the United States about discount calling services. People in the United States often receive bargain rates on telephone cards from their telephone company or membership-only clubs. The differences in price can be phenomenal.

To find out about discounts on calls to your home country, talk to those acquaintances from your own country who are in the United States. If you do not know anyone in the United States, try going to an ethnic store that serves immigrants from your country. If available, buy a newspaper that circulates among people of your ethnic group. Here, you should be able to find ads for bargain prices on calling cards that can be used to make calls to your country.

Keeping the lines of communication open while you are traveling in the United States will minimize anxiety for you as well as the people back home. It is not very expensive to do so if you know where to shop.

Where to Stay?

Most of the programs you apply to will send a list of hotels in their vicinity. As a rule, these will be slightly more expensive than what you could find on your own by doing a bit of research. One way is to become a member of a travel club such as the Automobile Association of America (AAA); this organization can provide you with all the necessary information about any area, free of charge, and you may be able to find a reasonably priced hotel or motel nearby. Another way is to see whether any of the economically priced motel chains are located in the area. Many such motel chains have branches all over the United States. Most of them also have a toll-free number that you can use to inquire about branches in specific locations. If you do not have the phone numbers for these chains, you can call the toll-free directory at 800-555-1212 (from within the United States) and ask for the number of any motel chain by name.

A telephone call within the United States made to a toll-free number results in no charge to the caller.

Traveling in the City

Ground transportation in the area you travel to may be very expensive. Some cities like New York are well connected by subways and buses. In cities that are not well connected by public transport, it may be more economical to rent a car. You should do this only if you feel confident driving here. My enquiries to several major car rental agencies have revealed that international drivers must fulfill three requirements before renting a car in the United States: (1) They should be at least 18 or 25 years of age (depending on different state laws in the United States), (2) They should have a valid driving license (try to get an international license while in your own country), and (3) They should have a major credit card.

THE INTERVIEW DAY

Being called for an interview means that your initial sales pitch has worked. You have succeeded in stirring the PD's interest enough that he or she wants to meet you in person. From here on, you have as much of a chance of being accepted into the residency program as any other interviewee. This holds true even in the case of the so-called courtesy interview. This is an interview call that a PD grants to a candidate not on the basis of the merit of his or her application but as a way of obliging someone he or she knows. For example, one of the colleagues of a PD might request that she call Dr. X for an interview. The PD does not feel that Dr. X deserves an interview call on the basis of his application alone, but she also does not want her colleague to think that she ignored the recommendation completely. So she asks the candidate to come for an interview as a courtesy to her colleague. Many people think such interviews are granted with no real intention to hire these candidates, but I have seen many candidates getting residency on the basis of a so-called courtesy interview. For any interview call, you should be ready to go in and do your best to accomplish your goal: gaining acceptance into the program.

Before I touch on some simple interviewing techniques that are readily available in any book on this subject, there are certain points I want to emphasize that are unique to IMGs. Some interviewers may have a stereotypical impression of people of your nationality or ethnic origin. You must demonstrate the ability to speak comprehensible English as well as to understand the language. Additional tips in this regard are given in Table 9–4.

Questions You May Be Asked

You should think carefully about the best possible answers to commonly asked interview questions. You do not necessarily have to say what you think the interviewee wants to hear.

The style of interviewing in the United States is generally casual and nonthreatening. The questions asked are the ones that can be answered in the form of a discussion rather than with a single right or wrong answer. You should be familiar with the following frequently asked questions and should practice your answers to avoid being thrown off balance during the interview.

- *"What do you think is your greatest strength?"* Think about this carefully and try to come up with an answer that makes an effective statement about you without sounding too pretentious.

TABLE 9–4. Special Interviewing Tips for IMGs

1. Wear conventional business attire. For men, this should be in the form of a dark suit, white shirt, and a conservative tie. For women, it could be in the form of a dark suit or skirt. Female candidates who do not feel comfortable in pants or a skirt should wear clothes that merge into the surrounding ambiance as much as possible. I feel the need to say all this because many IMGs have an impression of Americans as highly informal people. We may visualize them working in offices in shorts and Hawaiian shirts. This is a misconception. For one thing, America is a fairly conservative country, contrary to the expectations of the outside world. For another, people who are interviewing for a responsible position such as that of a physician are required to demonstrate a certain degree of conventionalism.
2. As an appendage to previous point, try to act according to the well-established norms of United States society. For example, I do not think the interview is the time to try to make a statement by wearing your ethnic or national dress. This is my personal view, and I do not want to offend anyone's feelings by saying so. On the other hand, if there are certain things that are part of your religious or cultural beliefs, stick to them. Most people will respect the person with the courage of his or her convictions.
3. At the other end of the pendulum, some IMGs may try too hard to act "very American." I think it is easier to understand an Indian being very Indian or a Pakistani being very Pakistani than either of them trying hard (unsuccessfully) to be an American. Just follow the rules that hold true in every corner of the world: Be charming, courteous, honest, and well turned out. You should look enthusiastic about the prospects of working as a resident. While you are doing all that, you should also keep selling yourself by talking about your strong points in a matter-of-fact way.
4. Counter to whatever you may have heard about work culture in the United States, you should not presume you are on a first-name basis with anyone unless that person requests that you use his or her first name. Address everyone by last name preceded by the appropriate title (e.g., Mr., Mrs., Ms., or Dr.). On the other hand, when introducing yourself, use your full name (first and last) without the title of Dr.
5. If you are a smoker, try not to smoke on the day of your interviews. If you cannot do that, avoid smoking in an enclosed space, as the smell of the cigarettes tends to stay on your clothes. This can be a real turn off to people who meet you. As a matter of fact, once you have smoked at all, it is quite a chore to deodorize yourself completely. The best tip of all? Quit smoking!
6. On the day of the interview, be pleasant to everyone—even the people who do not appear to be directly interviewing you. At some places, the secretaries and other ancillary staff can make a difference in your chances of being accepted into the program.

- ❑ *"What do you think is your greatest weakness?"* Use the answer to this question to show that you are aware of your imperfections. I suggest avoiding overused and tired answers such as "I am a perfectionist" or "I work too hard."
- ❑ *"Why did you apply to this program?"* The real reason you applied may be that the program is located in a city where you have a friend who was ready to provide you free room and board. At least that was a big consideration for me when I went on interviews. But you should do some research into each program to find out its strong points, and enumerate them in your answer.

- *"Why do you want to train here?"* The same advice holds true here, as well.
- *"Tell me about yourself."* This is an excellent opportunity for you to give a short presentation about yourself. Carefully prepare a summary of the things you want to say. Remember, you are a salesperson now trying to sell a product—you. Each sentence should be carefully crafted to clinch the deal. You have to be innovative and a bit of a psychologist here. Imagine what the person on the other side of the table expects you to be. I know that salesmanship is not a subject taught in medical school, but you have been in similar situations many times before. Remember those representatives from medical companies who came to you to sell their products? If they came to introduce a new drug, they knew they were competing with many other products in the same class. So, they always started with a statement that they thought would be likely to get you interested right from the start. Your presentation should follow a similar strategy. Prepare your answer to this question carefully and discuss it with others to see how it "plays".

Finally, you should read over your personal statement and CV carefully and be able to explain each statement or expand on the information given there.

Questions to Ask

There are lots of questions you may want to ask about a program. The interviewers can answer these. You should also try to talk to some current residents; they will often give you the most useful and honest answers to your questions. Some programs encourage interviewees to talk with their residents and interns. This could be in the form of lunch with the house staff or an after-interview dinner at a restaurant. Other places avoid this. At such places, the interviewees may receive an impression of well-orchestrated chaos. It may seem that they "somehow missed" meeting the house staff. Regard such programs with suspicion. As far as asking the relevant questions is concerned, I have found the following problems to be unique to IMG candidates:

- Most of the time, IMGs do not know the questions to ask.
- If they do know, they are often afraid to ask them, fearing that it may make them look too demanding. As long as you ask questions in a pleasant way, you have nothing to worry about. Interviewers always respect an informed candidate.

- ❑ If IMGs happen to be in the same interview group as U.S. medical graduates, they often do not seem to understand the importance of the questions asked by the American graduates. For instance, they may not understand slang terms such as "scut."

Here are a few tips that should help:

Do not ask the administrator of a residency program whether the program will sponsor you for a J-1 visa. Some PDs who are not used to the INS lingo may be scared off and say no. Keep in mind that the residency program does not sponsor you for the J-1 visa, ECFMG does.

1. If you are seeking to do residency on an H-1 visa, ask directly whether the program sponsors residents for this visa. Administrators of programs that have not had many IMG residents may have a tendency to say no as a first reaction. This arises out of the fear of the paperwork, and the unknown. You may have to do a bit of work to educate these people about what is actually involved.
2. Scut work: This is slang for the type of work that you should not have to do as a part of medical training—but that you end up doing anyway in some programs. Examples include residents having to transport patients, or having to draw blood samples for laboratory studies rather than having a phlebotomist draw them. These activities may seem small, but they can break the back of an already tired intern or resident. The importance of having sufficient support staff to fulfill these functions is underlined by the fact the regulating bodies such as the Residency Review Committee (RRC) and Accreditation Committee for Graduate Medical Education (ACGME) insist on such requirements for the continued accreditation of a residency program.
3. Ask about the different hospitals you may have to rotate through during your residency in a particular program. Find out the distance between different hospitals. Ask the current residents where they live and how far they travel, on average, on a daily basis. It is important to be as near to the workplace as possible. You will appreciate every extra minute of sleep you can get in the morning during the tiring days of your residency.
4. While collecting information, try talking to a resident who is in the same situation as you. For instance, only a person with children can give you a good idea about the quality of schools in the area. On the other hand, if you are single, a single person's perspective will be more important to you.

5. Call schedule: On average, programs require residents to be on call one in every four nights. They should let you go home a little early on a postcall day. See if this is the case. There is also supposed to be a cap on the number of new patients admitted by an intern in a 24-hour period; the maximum is five patients. See if the program follows that policy. Ask what the on-call day is like. What are your chances of getting some sleep on an on-call day? It should be possible to get some sleep in a well-managed program.
6. Some good programs give their residents time off for research. A good program should have a history of encouraging its house staff to go to conferences, with their main expenses paid.
7. The percentage of graduating residents passing the board certification examination is supposed to be a reflection of the quality of teaching in the program. I think it could also be a reflection of the instincts of the PD in choosing the right residents (e.g., those who are good exam-takers) for training. Anyway, it is nice to know this number. You can find out the percentage for each program by going to the Web site for FREIDA, listed earlier in the chapter.
8. While talking to the residents, find out what happened to the recent groups of graduating residents. See how many got into fellowships at desirable institutions and how many got the jobs they wanted. This in itself is a good summary statement of the performance of the program as a whole.
9. The preceding questions should be asked in a smooth conversational style. While trying to get answers to your questions, be courteous to the other interviewees and let them ask their questions. Oftentimes the questions they ask may be the ones that you were going to ask.
10. Ask questions that show your genuine interest in the line of training as well as that particular program. A little research done beforehand may give you lots to talk about here.

FOLLOW UP

After the interview is over, take some time—the same evening if possible—to jot down good and bad points about that program. You can use this checklist later to help you in ranking the programs.

Next, write a follow-up letter to the interviewers. To personalize it, you should try to write about a particular aspect of your conversation with that person. You can send this letter by e-mail, but you should also send it by conventional mail. These letters usually go into your file and may refresh the interviewer's memory of you when your file is reviewed at the time of ranking.

THE NEXT STEP

After all of your interviews have been completed, you should get ready for the NRMP match. Perhaps you are one of those people who is ready to go back to the home country after finishing the interviews. If so, now may be the time to do some shopping for the people back home.

CHAPTER 10

Building Your Nest

There is a lot of difference between coming to the United States on a tourist visa and coming to live here for a while. Once you are here, you have literally moved your home. You need a place to stay, a mode of transportation, a school for your child (if you have one), and much more. Just moving from one city to another can be a stressful event. But now you are moving to a country with a system that is entirely different from the one you are used to. Most of us have not even thought of these problems before coming here. I hope this book is of some help in this regard.

The process of settling in can be easier if you spend some time in the United States before you begin your residency program. Once you begin the residency, even simple—but usually more important—things will tend to be postponed forever. Try to arrive in the United States a few weeks in advance and take care of the items discussed below. Even if you arrive after the session has begun, take some time off to take care of these essentials before you begin your residency.

GETTING A SOCIAL SECURITY NUMBER

You need to obtain a Social Security number (SSN) before becoming employed. The SSN is also necessary for tax purposes, to receive general public assistance, and to obtain a driver's license and motor vehicle registration. Getting the SSN is an important first step before you can start your career in the United States. Your employer will need this number to put you on the payroll. You will be asked for this number whenever you close a major deal, including buying a car, getting loan, renting an apartment, and so on. Because it takes about 2 to 3 weeks for your request to be processed, this should be one of the first things you do after your arrival in the United States.

Getting a SSN should be one of the first things you do after arriving in the United States.

You can get information about the application for an SSN by calling toll-free 800-772-1213. It can be difficult to get through on this number, but I found that people handling these calls are very courteous and helpful. They can also provide you with information regarding the Social Security office nearest to you. When I called, the person I spoke with was even able to give me directions to the site over the phone.

You can also visit the Social Security Administration Web site at *www.ssa.gov*, where you can download application forms. However, it may be helpful to go to the office and complete the paperwork with the help of an official there.

According to the Social Security Administration Web site, the documents required to obtain a SSN are as follows:

1. Original documents showing your age and identity. Your passport should serve that purpose.
2. Original proof of lawful alien status. This could be in the form of an I-94 form or the visa stamp on your passport, your IAP, or any other paper relevant to your visa type.
3. The Web site states that you should "provide a letter on letterhead stationary from the government agency requiring you to get a SSN. . . ." In your case, your visa type should be self-explanatory as it indicates that you are here to work. The contract from your hospital may be another document that meets this requirement. Ask the Social Security Administration officials if they will accept some other form of evidence.

SSN FOR YOUR SPOUSE

Sometimes the Social Security Administration officials will ask you why you need an SSN for your spouse. Explain that he or she will need it to obtain a driver's license.

SSN FOR YOUR CHILDREN

According to the Social Security Administration Web site, a family member of the lawfully admitted alien does not need a SSN to:

- ❑ Register for school
- ❑ Report group health insurance coverage
- ❑ Apply for the school lunch program. For this, you need to get a letter from the Social Security Administration indicating that an SSN will not be assigned to your child.

However, nearly all IMGs feel more comfortable having an SSN for their children. Visit the Social Security Administration office and talk to the officials. Explaining why you want the SSN for your child can usually help expedite your request.

A THING CALLED CREDIT HISTORY

You will hear the term "credit history" within a few days of arriving in the United States. In the United States, virtually all major purchases are made on credit. People buy commodities and pay for them over the next few months. During the time that you live here, you will acquire a history of taking credits and paying them off. Credit rating agencies keep track of peoples' credit histories. If you pay your debts on time, you will have a good credit history. If not, it will be reported to these agencies. Every time you do anything that involves a credit reference, your credit history will be checked. If your credit history is bad, the creditor may be hesitant to give you any more credit.

Being new in this country, you have no credit history. You may be told by car dealers and landlords that you are not a good risk because you do not have a credit history. This is done to prevent you from bargaining for a good price. Do not let this scare you. First of all, to modify a common saying in the United States, no history is good history. Second, having a contract for residency in your hand makes you a good risk client.

FINDING A PLACE TO LIVE

Finding a place to live will be one of your biggest concerns. Following are a few helpful hints:

- Talk to the residents in your program to find out where they live. Having worked in the same hospitals for a year or more, they should have learned the good and bad points of living in a particular area. You can benefit from their experience.
- Discussions about different residential areas will also give you an idea about the safety of those areas. It is very important to be aware of the crime history of an area. In some cities, a crime-infested area may be only one street away from a safe area. It is important to know this before you become the prisoner of a legally watertight lease.
- Living in the same general area as your colleagues may provide much-needed social and emotional support to you and your family.
- Some apartments offer a monetary incentive to people who refer new tenants to them. If so, discuss the incentive with a friend and ask to use his or her name as the referring person. You can share the money or, better still, your friend may let you have it all.
- Do not sign a lease unless you are totally satisfied. If possible, take along someone who has been in the United States a little longer than you to look at the apartment and review the lease. Read through the lease carefully before signing and be sure you understand its terms.
- *Yes, there are cockroaches in America and a lot of other imperfections, too.* Look over the apartment carefully before you rent. If the carpet is dirty or the plumbing does not work, point it out to the landlord and ask that the problems be corrected. If you see even one cockroach in your apartment, you can be sure there will be thousands lining up for the food you will cook or eat in your new home. Keep in mind that once you sign the lease, even problems that were already present, but not noted in the lease, may be considered to have begun after you moved in. Be sure to report any problems you notice *before* signing the lease. Most apartment owners will look for damages to the apartment before returning the money you left as a security deposit at the end of your lease. Avoid giving them a free pass to your hard-earned money.

OBTAINING A DRIVER'S LICENSE

You can drive around for awhile in the United States with an international license. But you and, if married, your spouse should try to get a

U.S. driver's license as soon as possible. You may be able to move around easily using public transportation if you are in a city like New York, but in most cities you will want to have a vehicle of your own. It is very important that your spouse get a license, too. Even if he or she is not working, having some mobility will help maintain his or her sanity.

For instructions about how to get a license, you should get in touch with the secretary of state for your state of residence. As a general rule, you will need to have the following items:

- ❑ Your passport.
- ❑ Proof of residence in that state. This could be in the form of a utility bill or an apartment lease. If you are still living temporarily with someone, you can post a letter in your own name to the address where you live. This envelope with the post office stamp can act as a proof of residence for you.
- ❑ A Social Security Number
- ❑ A car to use during the driving test. If you do not have a friend who can lend you a car, you can usually pay a driving school to use one.

ARRANGING FOR TELEPHONE SERVICE

To arrange telephone service, you have to choose both a "local carrier" and a "long-distance carrier." The local carrier is responsible for calls in your immediate area; the other carrier handles your calls to other localities, states, and countries. You may have a choice of more than one local company in some locations. You will also have to choose a long-distance carrier. Typically most IMGs make hundreds of dollars worth of calls during their first few homesick months after arrival in the United States. This is also the time when they are usually paying extremely high rates for calls back home. Make a few calls to different service providers and shop around to find the best calling rates to your country. While discussing rates with different phone service companies, ask about the following points:

- ❑ Will you be charged the same low rate for the calls to your country seven days a week and at all times of the day or is the rate lower only on weekends and during specific hours of the day? The same questions should be asked regarding interstate calling rates within the United States.
- ❑ Will you have to pay extra every month to be able to get the quoted rate?
- ❑ How long will the quoted rate last? After this period, you may have to pay a much higher rate.

GETTING YOUR WHEELS

You have an enormous variety of car brands to choose from in the United States and haggling is the norm at automobile dealerships. You will have to decide whether to buy a new or used car. Again, ask the people you know what has worked for them. You may have difficulty initially in getting a loan to buy a car. Try the credit union of your hospital. If you do get stuck with a high-interest loan for a while, keep shopping around for a lower interest loan that you can use to pay off the higher interest loan.

LINING UP CAR INSURANCE

Car insurance in the United States is very expensive. As a new driver in this country, you have to pay a very high premium. Some big companies will not even offer you car insurance unless you have been driving in this country for at least 2 years. Others who may be ready to give you insurance at a *reasonable* premium may provide shameful service. You will probably have to strike a balance between the two. Try to find a reasonably dependable company that will not eat up too much of your paycheck each month.

Avoid buying unnecessary frills that may be offered by insurance agents. In some cases, these may repeat services you already have. For example, there is no point in buying roadside assistance if you are already a member of AAA. Some medical coverage may already be provided by your medical insurance carrier. This advice may save you some money.

OPENING A BANK ACCOUNT

The banking system in the United States is different from that of many other countries. You may be given a choice of several different types of accounts. You should choose the one that best suits your needs.

- ❑ Try to pick an account that does not impose large penalties if you fall below the minimum required balance.
- ❑ A basic checking account does not pay any interest, while a savings account pays a small percentage of interest. Many banks also offer interest-earning checking accounts, but these generally require you to maintain a large minimum balance.
- ❑ Choose an account that allows you to write enough checks per month to meet your needs without incurring any penalties.
- ❑ Open an account with a financial institution that is also ready to give you low-interest loan to buy a car or to meet other short-term needs. Small local credit unions sometimes offer the best deals.

ENROLLING IN A HEALTH INSURANCE PLAN

It is very important to buy a health insurance plan in the United States. The phenomenal cost of health care here makes it almost impossible to be able to pay out of pocket for more than the occasional health problem. One single serious problem can often wipe out a person's savings. If you are coming to the United States to join a residency program, your employer will offer you some kind of health insurance. You may not have much of a choice as far as the type of insurance you are offered. But it is very important that you understand the various terms used to describe these plans. I strongly recommend you read a booklet published by the Agency for Health Care Policy and Research entitled *Your Guide to Choosing Quality Health Care*. You can download it by going to their Web site at *www.ahcpr.gov* or can get it by calling 800-358-9295 (within the United States) or 410-381-3150 (outside the United States).

It is important to keep the following points in mind:

- Do be sure to enroll your dependents in your health plan. If they come to the United States after you, add their names as soon as possible after their arrival. If you do not do this within a given time, your dependents may not be covered by the insurance policy at all.
- Dental insurance needs to be purchased separately from regular health insurance.
- Different plans may not cover you for a specific time period (usually one to three months) after enrollment in the plan. Be aware of these gaps in coverage.
- If you have not had to pay a doctor for your own or your family's care since entering medical school because of prevalent professional courtesy in your own country, be ready for a rude awakening. Professional courtesy is almost nonexistent in U.S. medical circles.

FINDING YOUR COMPATRIOTS

Try to meet some people from your own country or ethnic group. These people may be able to tell you where to shop for food that you like. You may be able to find a place of worship or other places frequented by people of your own nationality or ethnic group. Some groups publish their own newspapers which can give you insights into the local community. This is more likely to be the case in larger cities like Chicago, New York City, or San Francisco.

GETTING TO KNOW YOUR TOWN OR CITY

As previously noted, United States cities can have an enormously mixed complexion. One area may be well-kept and crime-free while an adjoining area is dangerous. Be sure you know the general area well before heading out to explore your new neighborhood.

HITTING THE GLASS CEILING: HOW REAL, HOW MYTHICAL?

Once in the United States, it is all too easy to blame your little debacles on racism. I think America is still one of the most tolerant societies in the world. It may just take a little bit more work to reach the goals you aim for.

The United States also, has its own versatile definition of intelligence. This may frustrate some people who see some IMG colleagues with inferior academic records doing much better after arriving here. The explanation is that the United States does not have straightjacket criteria for "good" performance. Excellent public relations skills can take one far in the academic arena even if one is not exactly a genius in the traditional sense of the word. This phenomenon also prompts some purists from other countries to say that only mediocre individuals from other countries come to the United States. However, the tangible fact is that the people of the United States help to make it one of the greatest nations in the world.

CHAPTER 11

Survival Skills

YOUR FIRST MONTH OF RESIDENCY

Before starting work as a resident, you should have several books to keep at hand for quick reference. Most United States graduates carry these in their white coat pocket. Helpful books include the following:

1. Gilbert D, Moellering R Jr., Sande MA: *The Sanford Guide to antimicrobial therapy*, 29th ed., Hyde Park, VT: Antimicrobial Therapy, Inc., 1999.
   Address: P.O. Box 70, 229 Main Street
   Hyde Park, VT 05655
   Tel: 802-888-2855
   This book is published each year. It gives the antimicrobial drug of choice for various infections enumerated alphabetically. It also gives the list of antimicrobials that need dose adjustment for renal or hepatic impairment. The list of antimicrobials and their spectrum is provided in a tabulated form. It is a small, easy to carry book—"must have."
2. Di'Gregorio G, Barbieri E: *Handbook of commonly prescribed drugs*, 14th ed. Westchester, PA: Medical Surveillance, Inc., 1999.
   Address: P.O. Box 1629, West Chester, PA
   This book lists commonly used medicines in tabulated form, as follows: generic name, common trade name, therapeutic category, preparation (e.g., 100-mg tablet, inj. 5 mg/ml), and common adult dosage. This book does not give any side effects or interactions of various drugs. The size of the book is big in relation to the purpose it serves.

3. Green S: *The 1999 Tarascon pocket pharmacopoeia,* 1999 ed. Tarascon Press, 1999.
   This is a pocket-sized book giving medicines according to the system they act on. For each medicine the following information is given: generic name, common trade name, dose, dispensed dosages, prominent side effects, route of metabolism, safety in pregnancy or lactation, and whether the drug is DEA (Drug Enforcement Agency) controlled—an extremely useful book.
4. Ferri F: *Practical guide to the care of the medical patient,* 4rd ed. St. Louis: Mosby-Year Book, 1999.
   This book gives a concise and comprehensive account of commonly encountered clinical situations in an understandable format. This can be a useful companion on the floor.
5. Carey C, Lee H, Woeltje K: *The Washington manual of medical therapeutics,* 29th ed., Philadelphia: Lippincott-Raven, 1998.
   This is a very popular book with a format somewhat similar to that of Ferri, listed above.
6. The electronic diary comes in the form of a small palm-top computer. You can attach different cartridges to it—for example, attach a cartridge with *Harrison's*—and pull up brief notes on any topic of interest. This is quite useful for the computer-savvy resident.

The first month of residency is very stressful for everyone, but it can be an especially trying experience for IMGs. Most of us have not had a chance to get acquainted with the U.S. medical system as a student or otherwise. Rather than having a gradual increase of responsibilities, most interns undergo an abrupt immersion. The first time you enter a U.S. hospital as an intern, you will be expected to perform all of the intern's duties. You will have to work in a system that may be very different from the one you are trained in. Most IMGs have to communicate with an unfamiliar patient population, while speaking a language that is not their first language. Some programs have a system in place whereby seniors slowly induct interns into frontline duties. In others, the interns are more or less dropped into the middle of the action. The following pointers can help smooth your induction into a U.S. residency.

1. In contrast to the system in some other countries, most of the hospitals training residents in the United States are not totally funded by the government. The teachers or attending physicians in the hospital are also private practitioners. Their money comes from the regular stream of satisfied patients. Once you become an intern, you are a very important member of their service chain. This is different from your student days, when you were in the hospital only to learn and were never responsible for any business. This is also very different from the system of residency in some parts of the world, where residents are allowed to see patients at leisure and to study. In such situations, residents are not responsible for the business side of patient care.
2. The United States is a very litigious society. The danger of being sued by a dissatisfied patient is an everyday reality for physicians in the United States. A physician can be sued by a patient many years after his or her contact with that patient. The documentation in the patient's chart is the only record a hospital or physician has of the care provided to the patient years ago. This is the reason that you will find most people very particular about ensuring written documentation of all steps of care in the patient's chart. As a member of the team, your note could be a topic for discussion in a court of law one day. You will endear yourself to your seniors if you write sensible and complete notes for your patients.
3. For the reason cited above, every single step in patient care involves elaborate paperwork. This requirement can seem overwhelming in the initial weeks and months of residency. You must understand, however, that this paperwork is carefully constructed to protect you and your hospital. Some paperwork is designed to help the hospital bill for the services provided. The better programs should familiarize their interns with the common paperwork during the orientation period. If not, you should request one of your seniors or your chief resident to show you the most frequently used forms. Following is a list of paperwork you must be familiar with before you hit the floor:

   a. *H & P* (history and physical examination) *form:* This is the form you have to complete after initial assessment of every new patient in the clinic, emergency department (ED), or hospital. Some hospitals have a preprinted format in which you fill in the findings of your assessment. Others have a plain sheet on which you write the H&P according to a standard format, as described later in Chapter 12.

b. *Order form:* This is the form on which you write all of the orders, using a standard format. The format followed in U.S. hospitals can be remembered using the popular mnemonic ADC VAAN DISML.

A—Admit: Specify the admitting instructions; for example, "Admit on fourth floor under Dr. X, neurology service."
D—Diagnosis: Write the diagnosis relevant to nursing care. This should be the diagnosis or diagnoses that is/are the main reason for admission at this time.
C—Condition: Write "stable," "guarded," or "critical" as appropriate.
V—Vitals: Write the instructions about how frequently the vital signs should be recorded by the nurse. If you have no special orders, write "per protocol."
A—Activity: Indicate the activity allowed, namely "bed rest," "bathroom privileges," or "as tolerated," according to the patient's condition.
A—Allergies: Enumerate the drugs or other substances to which the patient is allergic. NKDA is the abbreviation used for "no known drug allergy."
N—Nursing: This is the place for issuing special instructions regarding any nursing care requirement that is unique to the given patient; for example, "strict intake–output charting," "sit the patient up in the chair twice daily," and so on.
D—Diet: Indicate the type of diet recommended for the patient; for example, "regular diet," "2 g sodium diet," "NPO" (meaning nothing by mouth), "2000-calorie ADA diet" (ADA stands for American Dietetic Association), and so on.
I—Intravenous fluids: Indicate the type of and the rate of infusion of the fluid to be given. If the patient does not need fluids, write "heplock," which indicates that the peripheral intravenous line should be inserted and should be kept patent by intermittent heparin flush.
S—Sedatives and analgesics.
M—Medications: This should include the dose, route, and frequency of administration:
L—Laboratory tests: These and other diagnostic studies should be ordered here. You should also specify when you want a particular test to be done.

c. *Prescription writing:* In the United States, most medicines are available only by prescription, when the patient presents a prescription written by a qualified doctor to a pharmacy. The prescription slip is a printed paper with the following components:

(1) The top portion has the name of the doctor(s) and a space for writing the date.

(2) There is a space for writing the name, age, and address of the patient.

(3) Under this, there is a blank space for writing the prescription information. On the first line, you should write the name of medicine: the next line should give the number of tablets or caplets or vials to be dispensed; the third line should have the dose, route of administration, frequency, and any other special instructions for taking the medicine.

(4) In the lower right-hand corner is a place for your signature, where you should also indicate if it is acceptable for the pharmacy to substitute a generic for a brand name drug. The lower left-hand corner has a box for specifying the number of refills. A refill allows the patient to get new supply of medicines once the original supply is finished. For the convenience of patients with chronic diseases, you will usually give many refills, whereas you probably will not give multiple refills to patients receiving antibiotic or controlled drugs. A sample of the main body of a prescription form follows:

XXX Clinic

Date ____________

Name Age ____________

Cap Amoxycillin 500 mg

#15

Sig: one capsule by mouth three times daily × 5 days

Refills: ☐ Times Signature ____________________

Product Selection Permitted

____

Dispense As Written

d. *Consent form:* This is a very important document. Some hospitals provide preprinted consent forms for the most commonly performed procedures which enumerate the risks and benefits of that procedure. This can make your job easier as you can read off the risks and benefits to the patient from this sheet. A person performing or assisting with the proposed procedure should obtain the consent to ensure that the patient receives an accurate account of the risks and benefits of the procedure. Oftentimes, however, interns are asked to obtain consent for a procedure they may be unfamiliar with. This can be a dangerous practice, as an inaccurate or inadequate explanation of a procedure places both the patient and the hospital (and staff) performing the procedure in a potentially litigious position. In the real world, of course, interns do have to obtain consent on others' behalf. If you are asked to do so, simply ask the senior resident about the risks that should be explained to the patient. Following are important points about the consent:

(1) Even if you provide the patient with a written consent form, the written text must be verbalized to the patient.

(2) A complete consent includes the name of the procedure, an explanation of how the procedure is performed, the benefits of the procedure, alternative modes of management in the absence of that procedure, and the risks of the procedure.

e. The forms for ordering various diagnostic investigations.

4. Good communication skills can spell the difference between glorious success and pitiful failure in the United States. I do not mean that you must have a flawless accent, but rather that you should be a sensitive person who knows the importance of communication with the patient and his or her family. You are tested on this aspect in the form of test items on the USMLE and also through the CSA. Various research studies in the United States have shown that the major cause of lawsuits in a physician's practice is lack or perceived lack of communication. Keep the following points in mind:

- Always inform the patient in advance about any investigations you are planning to schedule for him or her.
- If the patient's condition takes a turn for the worse, the family should be informed immediately.
- After you have seen a patient, you must discuss with the patient what you think about his or her problem. You do not have to pretend to know something you do not. Just discuss your plan to zero in on the diagnosis and management of the problem.
- If a mistake occurs in the care of the patient, the patient or family should be informed. In the initial stages of your training, you may want your seniors to handle such situations. If you do not quite know what is happening with the patient, concede ignorance. The key advice is to be honest and truthful.
- If a disagreement occurs between you and the patient or family, good communication and honest discussion is the only solution.
- While in the vicinity of the patient or in the overall work area of the hospital, never converse in your native language. This can prompt the people around you to guess at what you are saying, and it has landed many an IMG in trouble.

5. Patient confidentiality is a sacred concept in the United States. This concept holds that the information gained by you about a patient should never be shared with anyone else without the patient's consent. Some aspects of this concept are very commonsensical. Other aspects deserve special mention here:

   a. There may be situations where you may feel that your duty to maintain patient confidentiality clashes with your concern for someone else's safety. For example, informing the spouse of a patient about his newly detected HIV-positive status. In such cases, your initial effort should be toward convincing the patient to give this news to the spouse himself. This makes the matter so much simpler. In a different situation, if a patient expresses the desire to hurt someone, the doctor has a legal responsibility to make arrangements to inform the third party, ignoring the confidentiality.

   b. Even seemingly simple information about a patient's health should not be discussed with anyone else without the patient's consent.

6. Patient care in the office, ED, or inpatient setting is a team effort that involves numerous members. I discussed some of them in Chapter 8. Other important team members include:

   a. Social services: This is a very important component of the team. These individuals can help sort out many patient issues that have a social basis. People in the social service department are usually very resourceful. When in doubt, ask them if they can help with a particular problem. This can save you a lot of time.

   b. Pharmacists: They can provide guidance about the best antibiotic for a given bacterium or the right dosage of a drug or a particular side effect of a drug. Used judiciously, they can be an important help to you. But some of us from different training backgrounds feel uncomfortable about being "told" what to do with our patients by a pharmacist.

   c. Risk management: This department in a hospital provides guidance to hospital personnel about the legally safe techniques for dealing with different problems. This department, along with your teachers, should be informed promptly whenever you anticipate any legal problem arising out of the performance of your duties in the workplace.

   d. Home health: In many situations, a patient is not sick enough to require hospitalization but is still in need of medical care, for example, IV injections or regular wound dressings. Home health personnel can provide these services at the patient's home as required.

   e. Occupational and physical therapists (OT/PT) and speech therapists: The first two designations are self-explanatory; the speech therapist in addition to providing speech therapy evaluates the swallowing ability of patients. This may be an important consideration before initiating oral feeding in a patient after a stroke.

   f. Doctors on other services: Just as you are working with a particular service, there are residents, fellows, and attendings working in other departments. Don't forget to use this consulting resource when a perplexing problem happens to fall in the realm of another specialization.

USEFUL HINTS FOR SURVIVING THE FIRST MONTH

The first month of residency is a crucial period in your career. This is the period when lots of people are going to form opinions about you. You can very well (sometimes wrongly) be branded "lazy," "dishonest," "dumb," or "great" in the very first month of your internship.

- Equipped with the information given earlier, start your residency with full vigor and a positive attitude.
- Go in ready to work to your fullest potential. The qualities most appreciated in an intern are dependability and a willingness to work hard.
- Be all smiles. Remember that a tired but smiling person is more likely to get a helping hand than a bitter tired person.
- Project a positive attitude. Many IMGs may be "redoing" their internship, having completed a very high level of training in their own country. Never let this stand in the way of a good and courteous performance as an intern. If anything, this training should help you be a great intern, helping to endear you to other team members as a modest, intelligent person.
- When in doubt, ask the people who are likely to know better: nurses and significant others. They expect you to ask. Keep in mind that they see you as a complete novice and are as apprehensive working with you on the floors as you are working there.
- Nurses will sometimes, seemingly casually, run an important piece of information by you. Just because they do not emphasize it strongly, do not be lulled into doing nothing. Carefully evaluate each piece of information given to you. Whenever you are given information, ask the nurse what he or she thought should be done. Most nurses will tell you why they felt the need to call you. If you do not quite understand the significance of information given to you, ask your senior resident.
- If you order a test, you should follow the results, come what may. The burden of taking action according to the test result lies on the person ordering it. Some hospitals have a multitiered system of reporting abnormal laboratory test or other investigation results. But in the best of the facilities, things do fall through the cracks. If they do, it will be you who finds yourself under the axe.

- Once you think of a diagnosis, you should make arrangements to prove or disprove it. Apart from patient care issues, there is a serious liability issue here, too. There will be many situations where the attending physician, based on his or her experience will not agree with your diagnosis. It is still okay to write down your thought process and document the results of your discussion with your senior resident or your attending. In the end, proper documentation is good for the team as a whole.
- In the next section of this chapter, I will review several responses that should be on the tip of your tongue. The two phrases I am not including, but that should always be on the tip of your tongue are, "Thank you" and "Please."

FREQUENTLY ASKED QUESTIONS DURING AN ON-CALL DAY (OR NIGHT)

In the next part of this chapter, I present a systematic approach that you can use in dealing with the issues that most often necessitate calls to residents from nursing staff. Most of these questions will come in the form of pager calls when the resident or intern is busy carrying out other tasks such as admitting a patient. In such situations, it is essential to be able to judge the situation quickly and respond over the phone. Otherwise, the resident may have to physically run all over the place or, worse still, the patient may suffer because of delays or errors in judgment.

ACCUCHECK

This term refers to a common test for blood glucose level. Consider the following typical exchange:

Nurse: Doctor, Mr. Jones' blood glucose is 300.
Doctor: Is he a known diabetic?

This question is very important. Without knowing the answer, you might give insulin to the patient based on a wrong reading or patient mixup. If the answer is yes, ask whether the patient is on medication for diabetes.

Hyperglycemic Patient

If patient is not receiving medication for elevated blood glucose, you may decide not to give anything if the level is less than 300 mg/dl. If it is greater than 300, you should repeat the glucose levels. If more than 400, you should repeat immediately by accucheck machine as well as in the laboratory. If the level is still abnormal, treat. This policy may not be without controversy in certain situations. There is some literature suggesting that tight blood glucose control in the perioperative period may help wound healing. Research also suggests that better glucose control may improve the outcome in stroke patients. When in doubt, however, remember that slight hyperglycemia is safer than hypoglycemia, which can be fatal if undetected.

If the patient is on an oral hypoglycemic or antidiabetic drug and received a dose in the evening, you may decide not to take action if the blood glucose level at night is less than 300. Above that level, treat on its own merit.

If the patient received regular insulin more than 4 hours ago, determine the dose according to the present reading. If he got NPH insulin more than 8 hours ago, consider giving a dose of regular insulin. Keep in mind that NPH effects persist for almost 24 hours. If the glucose level is above 450, remember to order a ketone level and perform a mental status assessment.

It is important to discuss the target glucose levels with your team during regular rounds in the morning. This will give you confidence in managing diabetic patients and reduce your fear of being yelled at by the senior residents the next day.

The other way to avoid being called about accuchecks is to write a sliding scale. In this approach, you write an order for a dose of regular insulin to be given for a given blood glucose level, for example:

Accucheck Result (mg/dl)	Regular Insulin Subcutaneous
151–200	2 U
201–250	4 U
251–300	6 U
301–350	8 U
351–400	10 U
> 400	Call MD

I do not want to imply that this scale is the best or even the most popular available. It is included here simply to introduce you to the concept of the sliding scale.

Hypoglycemic Patient

What if the nurse tells you the patient's blood glucose level is less than 60? Ask about patient's mental status. If it is normal and the patient is able to swallow, give him juice or any sweet beverage to swallow (*not* an artificially sweetened beverage). If the patient has altered mentation, or the blood glucose level is less than 40, order 50% dextrose IV and rush to see the patient.

In either of these situations, do not forget to try to find the reason for the hypoglycemia or the very high glucose level and remember to modify the patient's medications as warranted. If an oral hypoglycemic agent is the cause of hypoglycemia, you will have to continue the dextrose infusion for a longer period.

HEPARIN AND COUMADIN ADJUSTMENT BASED ON PROTHROMBIN TIME (PT) AND PARTIAL THROMBOPLASTIN TIME (PTT)

Many patients receiving oral or parenteral anticoagulants will be under your care. You will be responsible for adjusting their dosages of heparin or Coumadin (warfarin) according to the results of PT/INR or PTT, respectively.

Adjusting Heparin

The low molecular weight heparin (LMWH) has made things much easier for interns and residents responding to floor calls. With LMWH, unlike the situation with IV heparin, you do not have to perform frequent PTTs. This means you do not get called in the middle of the night with the PTT results. I have seen a lot of research data that favorably compare LMWH with IV heparin in different disease conditions. If your patient is receiving heparin, you should be aware of the following issues of care:

- What is the target PTT? This may vary from lab to lab; moreover, the primary physician may set his or her own desired range according to a perception of the seriousness of the disease process or due to some other complicating factor.
- If the PTT was performed at least 4 to 6 hours after the initiation of an IV drip, and is near the baseline (e.g., 30 to 45), consider giving another bolus of 3000 to 5000 units IV heparin and increase the drip rate by 100 units per hour. Repeat the PTT 4 to 6 hours after the adjustment. If the PTT still falls short by up to 20 points, consider the same approach with the exception of giving the bolus.
- If the PTT is up to 50 points higher than the upper limit of the therapeutic range, consider decreasing the rate by 100 units an hour and repeat the PTT in 4 to 6 hours. If the PTT is still significantly beyond this level, consider stopping the heparin for an hour and restarting at 100 to 200 units less than the previous rate. Repeat the labs as suggested before.
- In all the cases, make sure that the blood sample is not drawn from the same line as the one with the heparin drip. Otherwise you will get a spuriously high reading. Draw the blood sample at least 4 to 6 hours after initiation or adjustment of the drip rate to allow necessary time for equilibration of the effect.

Adjusting Coumadin

Some of your patients may be receiving the oral anticoagulant Coumadin. The dosage of Coumadin needs to be adjusted in order to reach the desired level of INR. But before you decide about the dosage adjustment, you should know the indication for Coumadin in the particular patient. The desired INR may vary according to the indication for anticoagulation. Many physicians shoot for an INR of 2 to 3 in patients with atrial fibrillation and deep venous thrombosis (DVT). The desired INR may be 3 to 4 in cases of mechanical prosthetic valve. Some patients may be on fixed low-dose Coumadin regardless of the INR. Following are several points worth remembering:

- If a patient with a stable INR on a given dosage of Coumadin begins to show poor control of INR, look for the reason for this change. It could be an interaction with another drug or a change in patient's health status or dietary habits.

- You may face difficult situations in caring for patients receiving Coumadin. For example, your patient who is receiving Coumadin after a prosthetic valve replacement may develop GI bleeding or an intracranial hemorrhage. The first step of course will be to stop the Coumadin. You must also take definitive steps to treat the bleeding (if possible) as soon as possible, for example, cauterization of the bleeding vessel in the stomach. The decision to halt the Coumadin will be the easy one, but the cause of concern will be the function of the prosthetic valve without anticoagulation therapy. The approach here should be decided after discussion with the team. The literature suggests that you may be able to restart low-dose Coumadin even in a case of intracranial bleeding, depending on the concerns regarding the disease process that necessitates Coumadin administration.
- There may be conditions that necessitate anticoagulation therapy during pregnancy. There have been reports of teratogenic effects of Coumadin. The emergence of LMWH may provide an alternative method of anticoagulation therapy for pregnant women.
- The dosage of Coumadin may need to be adjusted in order to achieve an INR in the desired range. There is an enormous amount of research that has tried to predict a maintenance dosage of Coumadin based on some formulae or other factors. Additional research has compared empirical dosage adjustment with that according to a suggested scale. The different research shows evidence in favor of either of these two methods. Most hospitals have Coumadin clinics that are run by pharmacists who help with adjustment of Coumadin dosages. It may be helpful to talk to them about the protocol followed by your hospital.
- Excessive anticoagulation can be another problem. If the INR is high without any bleeding, you may manage it conservatively by adjusting the Coumadin dosage. If the need for reversing anticoagulation is emergent, you may use fresh frozen plasma (FFP). If you plan to use vitamin K, use only 2 to 3 mg/dose as bigger doses may overcorrect. This overcorrection in turn, may be detrimental to the condition demanding anticoagulation.

BLOOD PRESSURE

This is another area that residents are called about frequently. As a generic response, the resident or intern orders a singly dose of some antihypertensive medication that he or she likes. It makes the resident feel good, and the nurses are satisfied, but we may not have done any good to the patient. I call this response "blood pressure cosmetics," as it is an intervention taken to make the numbers look nice to us.

You should intervene to lower blood pressure in following conditions:

- If there is evidence of acute and end-organ damage; for example, pulmonary edema, chest pain, altered sensorium, intracranial bleeding, or acutely worsening renal function that can be attributed to hypertension.
- The BP is more than 190 mm Hg, the diastolic pressure is more than 110, and no antihypertensive medication has been prescribed for the patient. Even in such conditions, your goal does not have to be to bring the BP down to the ideal level within minutes. Do not use suglingual nifedipine for an acute BP "fix."

Other things to keep in mind are as follows:

- Do not attempt to aggressively lower the blood pressure in cases of ischemic stroke.
- When a high BP reading is noted, review the patient's antihypertensive medications to consider the duration of their effect.
- Rather than acting to correct every high BP reading, the previous day's data should be used to adjust patient's regular dose of antihypertensives.

PAIN KILLERS

Pain has been recognized to be a markedly ignored ailment. The reason could be that there is no objective method of quantifying and documenting this problem; thus, there are no scary numbers demanding to be fixed. You will frequently be called by the nurses because a patient is asking for a "pain pill." You must have the following information available before prescribing such pain medications over the phone:

- Make sure that the pain is not an indicator of some potentially serious problem such as ischemic limb, intracranial hemorrhage, angina, or ruptured viscous. A rough but in no way foolproof indicator of the benign nature of a problem includes a headache similar to the ones patient has had in the past, pain that is not relatively sudden and is not excruciating, and stable vital signs.
- If this is the same type of pain the patient has had in the past, ask what has worked before. Prescribe the same drug if you do not see any contraindications.
- Before prescribing a nonsteroidal antiinflammatory drug (NSAID), inquire about a history of renal insufficiency or peptic ulcer. Also keep in mind that medicines belonging to this group do somewhat nullify the effects of angiotension-converting enzyme (ACE) inhibitors.
- Before prescribing acetaminophen, enquire about a history of liver problems. Almost every American has grown up with Tylenol, a popular brand name for acetaminophen.
- In the absence of contraindications and if the severity of pain demands, do not hesitate to use analgesics with codeine, or medicines belonging to morphine group.

FEVER SPIKE

You need to know the following things if you are called about a patient with fever:

- Has the patient had a fever since his or her hospital admission? If the answer is yes, is he or she already receiving appropriate therapy for it? If yes again, you may not have to do anything further. If the patient is known to have fever and is not receiving therapy for it, you may want to see if the appropriate studies have been ordered.
- If this is the first time the patient has had a fever during this hospital visit, you may want to take a brief history and order tests such as blood cultures (two sets from two different sites), urine exam and culture, and chest X-ray, if appropriate. If the patient is immunocompromised or neutropenic, you should consider starting antibiotics empirically.

CHEST PAIN

- Ask about the co-morbid conditions because hypertension and diabetes are important risk factors for coronary artery disease (CAD). Moreover, if the patient was admitted with pneumonia and has been having pain on deep inspiration, this information may help in diagnosis.

- Ask the patient's age. This is an important risk factor.
- Is the patient known to have CAD, pneumonia, gastroesophageal reflux, or chest trauma?
- Is there any known reason for similar pain that has been documented in the past?
- Is there a history of fever, diaphoresis, or shortness of breath?
- If the patient has had similar pain in the past, what intervention(s) helped?
- Your threshold for ordering an ECG for a patient with chest pain should be very low. And when you order it, do not leave the patient until you have read it. If you have any doubt, show or fax it to the people who are supposed to know better.
- The character of the pain is very important. Be aware especially of patient reports of a feeling of constriction or feeling of weight on the chest. Patients with such complaints are more likely to have pain that is cardiac in origin. Ask the patient who has had documented angina in the past if the present pain is reminiscent of prior episodes. If the answer is yes, it is more than likely to be cardiac. It has been observed that every patient tends to have what I will call his or her "signature pain." Thus, the character of subsequent episodes of angina tends to be similar to the first episode.

PAINFUL ABDOMEN

Patients complaining of pain in the abdomen should always be treated with due respect. You should inquire about the severity of pain, nausea, or vomiting. In all cases, you must examine these patients for any sinister signs such as absent bowel sounds, rebound, or guarding.

NEW ADMISSION

One of the main responsibilities of an intern on call is taking care of the new admissions. This means obtaining the H&P information for these new admissions and writing orders. All of this is done with the help of the resident on call. A lot of times, you may be called for a new admission while you are still working on a patient who arrived on the floor a few minutes before. Sometimes, this can be an acid test of your team play and management skills. The following factors can make this scenario difficult to deal with:

- If there is poor teamwork between resident and intern, an admission day can become very stressful for both.
- There is always an element of possible surprise on any hospital floor. For example, you may decide to see the next admission about an hour after you have finished working up the previous patient. But the new patient may deteriorate suddenly in the intervening period. This possibility can cause you to run from place to place just to "eyeball" the new patients.
- To add a little to your hassle, you may be asked a bunch of questions about a new patient whom you have not yet laid eyes on. The types of questions raised by the nurses could be, "This is dinner time, what kind of diet can I order for Mr. X?" or "What can I give to Mr. Y for pain?"

Following are several helpful tips that can help you tackle the issues attached to a new admission.

Different Sources of Admission

1. Hospital emergency department admits: This is self-explanatory.
2. Direct admits: These are patients whose doctors asked that they be admitted to the hospital floor directly. These doctors have admitting privileges in your hospital. Some of these doctors are very good about calling one of the members of the admitting team and others are not. These admissions, when unannounced, can be aggravating as well as full of surprises.
3. Clinic admits: These patients are admitted after an attending physician in the outpatient clinic has seen them. These patients are admitted after their doctor has examined them. If the admitting doctor calls you about the admission, he or she should be able to tell you the precise reason for admission. Sometimes the patient is admitted without any working diagnosis but simply because the physician feels "uncomfortable" about the patient's condition. You should always trust the caring physician's hunch and get on with the business of trying to find out what is wrong with the patient. This particular subgroup of patients should be seen (even if briefly) as soon as they reach the floor.
4. Intrahospital transfer: Suppose a patient is admitted to the internal medicine service. During the hospital stay, she goes into respiratory failure. The intensive care unit (ICU) resident may be

called for a consult. After evaluating the patient, the resident decides to transfer the patient's care to the ICU service. This is an example of intrahospital transfer. Patients who are transferred are always seen by some member of your team, so you will have a pretty good idea of how urgently you need to rush to see them.

5. Transfer from another hospital: This type of patient is a potential land mine. These patients are transferred from another hospital after they are accepted by one of the physicians in your team. The only thing you know about the patient's condition is what your team members have been told by the people in another hospital. Sometimes that information may not come from the best of sources. Moreover, a lot may change while patient is en route to your hospital. These patients must be seen as soon as they enter your territory of responsibility.
6. Through regular admitting department: These patients are admitted electively for a purpose. You should be able to see them at your leisure unless they happen to develop a different complaint after being admitted.

This description is provided to help you prioritize your time properly as you try (in vain, of course) to do too many things at the same time.

Other Helpful Hints

- Whenever you are called for a new admission, ask for the patient's vital signs. This may be difficult as often the floor secretary will tell you about the new admission. Nevertheless, you have to insist that you be given this information. Insist on talking to the nurse. Ask how the patient looks. This is another hedge against the possibility that you will wait too long before seeing a very sick patient.
- If you cannot see a new admission anytime soon, tell the nurse to call you back if there is any problem with the new patient.
- Avoid giving orders for seemingly small things such as diet or pain killers for the patients you have not yet seen.

VOMITING

This is another reason for calls to residents in the middle of the night. Before you order an antiemetic, you should make sure you are not missing any potentially serious condition. Ask about the number of vomiting episodes, whether there is pain in the abdomen, and the character of the vomiting (e.g., green, bilious). If you are called about the same patient vomiting time and again, you must go see that patient rather than loading him or her with different antiemetics.

SLEEPING PILLS

Ask yourself the following questions before ordering a sleeping pill for a patient:

- ❑ Is the patient having any respiratory distress?
- ❑ Does the patient have any altered mental sensorium?
- ❑ Is there any history of liver failure?

Use caution in prescribing sleeping pills to patients belonging to above sub-groups and older patients.

"UNCOOPERATIVE" PATIENTS

If you receive a call about a patient who is "uncooperative," you must go see that patient. Oftentimes these patients have an as-yet-unidentified but life-threatening condition. Sometimes residents are pressured to prescribe restraints for these patients. Always examine such patients before prescribing restraints for these reasons: First, you may be ignoring something very serious that is going on with the patient. Second, it is inexcusable to restrain a human being without having a genuine reason for doing so. Do not leave the patient's bedside until you have made up your mind about the reason for patient's belligerence, abusiveness, or uncooperativeness.

"DEPRESSED" PATIENTS

This group of patients is another potential land mine. A person who looks depressed to a physician may in fact have a serious disease process that is responsible for his or her depressed demeanor. Always evaluate these patients carefully. If the diagnosis of depression is reasonably certain, you should make sure that the patient is not suicidal. A genuinely suicidal patient needs to be placed under one-to-one observation by an attendant in the hospital.

LEARNING TO FUNCTION AS A PUBLIC RELATIONS (PR) PERSON

One factor that makes the residency very tough is that you have to deal with so many different persons who are likely from different cultures. One tip to survival is to try to think what you would expect the other person to do if you two happened to trade places. Another tip is to try to study your colleagues' pet peeves. If things go wrong sometime nonetheless, and you see someone charging toward you, the best thing to do is to smile and listen. You may feel like a bit of a wimp for a while, but you will still be able to sleep at night, you will not have started another Cold War, and probably you will receive an apology from the aggressor in the very near future.

You will have to work with a new group of residents, interns, and attendings every month. By virtue of their different cultural backgrounds, these persons will be as diverse as any humans could possibly be. The ability to deal with these different human beings can make or break your future dreams. The problem is more profound for IMGs. Many of us do not realize the importance of these interpersonal relations. I have become fascinated with this topic as I have delved deeper into the importance of being a good PR person during residency in the United States. The next section provides some tips on how to deal with the different members of your team.

DEALING WITH THE MEMBERS OF YOUR TEAM

JUNIOR RESIDENT

According to the responses to a questionnaire given out by one of my colleagues, Dr. M. Makhsousi, to the senior residents, to be adjudged a good intern:

Do

. . . Be punctual, honest, respectful, and responsible.

. . . Keep your senior resident informed of all that is happening with your patients.

. . . Be a good team player.

Don't

. . . Lie. If you do not know something about your patient, go look it up and tell.

. . . Intervene if you are not sure

SENIOR RESIDENT

It is very important for the senior resident on a team to be on good terms with the junior members. On the basis of the responses to a second questionnaire given out to interns, to be adjudged a good senior resident:

Do

. . . Ask for the intern's input during the decision-making process. Give answers to questions when necessary.

. . . Be prepared to discuss a pressing issue regarding another patient even in the middle of rounds.

. . . Be calm and gentle when pointing out mistakes.

. . . Be the interns' advocate when appropriate.

Don't

. . . Make decisions without discussing them with the team.

. . . Get upset if a junior resident comes to you with a problem.

. . . Panic.

. . . Disappear when needed.

. . . Forget the end-of-rotation party (pun intended!).

CHIEF RESIDENT

A chief resident is a final-year resident or a person who has already finished his or her residency. The main activities of a chief resident include running the schedule for the residents and managing the teaching activities for the residents. It is possible for a chief resident to make a resident's life miserable. The first step toward finding a solution to any of your problems is to verbalize them. If you have a problem, you should talk to the chief resident about it. When you go in with a problem, you should suggest a solution as well. This increases your chances of being successful in resolving the problem to your satisfaction.

ATTENDING PHYSICIAN

Presenting a patient's case to the attending physician by phone can be a scary experience, especially in the beginning. A few of the common concerns and their suggested solutions follow.

- *Will the attending get mad at me if I call him or her at this time?*
  If there is a senior resident available, talk to that person first. Involve him or her in the decision to call the attending. This way, you can double-check the appropriateness of your call. Moreover the senior resident will also probably know how that particular attending is likely to respond.
- *What if the attending disagrees with you entirely?*
  The most important thing you need to remember is that you are in training. There should be no place for ego when it comes to the learning process. If you think a wrong decision is being made, you should discuss it with the attending physician.
- *How much information does the attending want?*
  Some attendings want full-length H&P and others want only the bare minimum. Worse still, the same attending may be ready to listen to pages worth of narrative one time and be abrupt and impatient the next. I think it is best to approach each patient presentation in the most professional and systematic way. That way, you will not miss any important points. You will be safer with this approach even if your attending is rushed for time. You will gradually understand the operating style of different attendings. These things do get better with time.

NURSES

Most IMGs will notice some important differences in the physician–nurse relationship in the United States as compared to that in their own country. The notable differences include the following:

- In some countries, the nurse may be a passive entity who simply carries out the orders given by a doctor. In the United States, the nurse is an equal member of the patient care team.
- In the litigious society of the United States, in the event of a lawsuit, nurses can be held equally responsible for a perceived mis-

take in patient care. This is why they may cross-check all of your orders and may tell you if they differ with you. Be respectful of their feedback. If you still think that your action is correct, discuss it with one of your seniors or colleagues. Sure there may be a rare nurse who will give you the runaround as part of his or her own ego trip. Nevertheless, you should strive to remain respectful and professional whenever you find yourself in this situation.

Do not let yourself be "psyched out" by all the gadgetry in the ICU. Knowing how to run those machines is a very small part of patient care.

SURVIVING THE ICU ROTATION

Being on call in the ICU can be a terrifying experience. From an IMG's perspective, the following aspects are most likely to cause you anxiety:

- This is an area with a lot of high-tech machinery that you may not know anything about.
- Your patient's condition may suddenly deteriorate and you may have to make split-second decisions.
- You may not know how to put in "lines"—this is slang for the central venous or peripheral arterial catheter insertions.

As any senior resident can tell, the ICU is not as complicated a place as you initially think. Following is some basic advice that can help make your life during the ICU rotation much easier.

- The ability to insert "lines" is not indispensable for your survival in the ICU. Even if your patient absolutely needs a central catheter, there will be plenty of help available to assist you.
- Do not let the machinery around the patient psych you out. Put all your training to use while managing the patient. There will always be staff members nearby who are supposed to know how to handle those machines.
- Your main thrust should be toward what I call "the fire fighting operation." In emergency situations, you have to maintain a focus on vital signs without going deeply into theoretical stuff. Follow the standard dictum of "ABC." A is the airway; this means the patient's airway should be cleared and opened by simple maneuvers such as the jaw thrust. B is for breathing; this can be assisted by using an ambu bag. You do not need to feel rushed to put in an endotracheal tube as long as enough air is getting into the patient's lungs. C is for circulation; this means you should keep the patient's blood pressure at a level adequate for perfusion. Fluids, blood products, or inotropes as deemed

appropriate can do this. Once these three things are taken care of, or while you are handling them, you can start the process of investigating the cause for the patient's unstable condition.

- Most acute patient conditions in the ICU can be handled using an algorithmic approach. The nurses are usually very helpful, and some of them will have years of experience behind them. Ask for and accept their help graciously.
- Most IMGs will recall several strange-looking questions on the USMLE 1 and 2. These are mostly in the form of "what will you do next?" The answers to such questions as related to cardiac emergencies come from the advanced cardiac life support (ACLS) literature. Most residency programs offer ACLS courses as a part of their orientation before new residents start the program. These courses teach a step-by-step approach to dealing with various cardiac emergencies. It is helpful to be thoroughly familiar with these steps when a patient's condition demands split-second decisions. I strongly recommend that you learn the ACLS protocols before taking the USMLE 2 and 3. Look for the ACLS booklet in your medical school library.

TABLE 11–1. Tips for Handling a Ventilator Problem

Note: Always call for the help of a more experienced person until you become very comfortable trouble shooting ventilator problems.

- Whenever the ventilator alarms go off and patient's respiratory status deteriorates, disconnect the patient from the ventilator and ventilate the patient with an ambu bag. This excludes one (machine) possible source of the problem.
- Whenever a patient on a ventilator develops sudden hypoxia, think pneumothorax or blocked endotracheal tube. Look for the typical signs of pneumothorax; increased resonance and decreased breath sounds. If suspicion is high, the threshold for putting a needle in the second intercoastal space in the parasternal area should be very low.
- As soon as possible, the goal should be to bring the FiO_2 back to < 0.6. This is needed to avoid O_2 toxicity.
- ABG abnormalities in a patient should always initially be treated as representative of some underlying disease process. All steps should be taken to address the precipitating factors.
- If ABGs indicated pH abnormality in the presence of normal PaO_2 or PCO_2, look for any process that could be responsible for this metabolic abnormality.
- To increase oxygenation, you can increase FiO_2, PEEP, or pressure support.
- To increase ventilation (lower high CO_2), increase the tidal volume or respiratory rate. The point to note here is that you should not put a patient on ventilator just to get the CO_2 into the normal range. Patients who have chronic high CO_2 should be intubated only if they have marked uncompensated metabolic acidosis or altered sensorium.
- There has been interest recently in noninvasive ventilation; this means assisting ventilation without putting an endotracheal tube down the patient's throat. This approach can be considered in a patient with respiratory failure who is expected to breathe adequately on his or her own.
- A BiPap mask is used during the night by patients with sleep apnea.

ABG, arterial blood gas; BiPap, Bilevel Positive Airway Pressure; PEEP, positive end-expiratory pressure.

- Ventilator scare: Most of us are very shaky about the management of ventilators. Apart from your senior residents, respiratory therapists can be a great help here. These are the technicians who are trained to handle the ventilators. In addition, familiarity with the actions outlined in table 11–1 should help to allay your anxiety.

DEALING WITH THE "UNEXPECTED"

These are situations that any normal human being can find himself or herself in; however, everyone has different expectations of a resident. That is why I am setting off the word "unexpected" in quotes here. Your main focus when dealing with such situations should be on describing the importance of the situation to your colleagues or senior staff members.

PREGNANCY DURING RESIDENCY

Fellow residents and other staff may grumble about a resident or intern becoming pregnant during the residency, but it is illegal to discriminate against a pregnant person under U.S. law. It is always good to let your colleagues know about your pregnancy far in advance of your expected date of delivery. This gives people time to prepare for the situation that will occur when the program is short by a resident.

ILLNESS

Do not ignore a health problem that is affecting you or your family. Yes, you have many important responsibilities as a resident, but your health and the health of your family should come first.

FAMILY EMERGENCIES

Some IMGs may have to deal with mishaps involving family members in their home country. If it is important that you fly back home, you should be able to say so to your program director.

ATTENDING CONFERENCES

The good programs always allow leave to their residents for educational activities. Some programs will pay for you to attend conferences and other academic meetings. The main problem with attending conferences is that you have to be able to leave without compromising your patient care responsibilities. This is possible if one of your colleagues is ready to take over your responsibilities or you are in a less busy (also called a "light") rotation.

* * *

One very real problem involves some residents who tell lies to stay away from work. It is essential that the people you work with have confidence in you as a responsible and conscientious person. "Unexpected" events are always handled more easily by persons judged to be trustworthy by their colleagues.

CHAPTER 12

Getting Through the Residency

HISTORY-TAKING, AMERICAN STYLE

History-taking is often described as being both an art and a science. It involves good interviewing techniques and a deep fund of knowledge of medicine. The ability to take a concise but complete history comes with knowledge and experience, which in turn is the result of hard work over the years. As a new doctor, you should focus on being systematic and thorough.

All of us have witnessed or heard about incidents in which an experienced physician made the right diagnosis on the basis of a few quick questions. Those are glorious examples of a good history-taking.

DEVELOPING THE ART

You should choose a good textbook on history-taking and physical examination. I am sure you have used such books during the medical school years. Go back to the same books and reread them with specific attention to the following areas:

- Interviewing techniques
- How to deal with "difficult" patients
- A systematic approach to the examination of each system
- The proper way to elicit different signs

Many other books are available that present differential diagnoses on the basis of symptoms. Still others offer guidelines on how to proceed with the history according to the patient's chief complaint. These books are all useful to read and digest.

One way of quickly accumulating knowledge is to read about a disease on the same day you see a patient with that disease. In this way, you will quickly add to your mental database. This approach will be useful to you throughout life. Let me give you an example. You see a patient with leg weakness who is found to have diabetic neuropathy. You read about this condition and find out that diabetic neuropathy can be painful. This gives you one differential diagnosis for any future patient complaining of leg weakness accompanied by pain. This is the best way of making yourself into a good clinician. There are certain common diseases that one comes across time and again during one's career as an internist. You should read about those diseases in one of the major textbooks.

In the next part of this chapter, I will emphasize some of the key aspects of history-taking, American style.

COMPONENTS OF THE HISTORY

Chief Complaints

This is why the patient has come to see you. As far as possible, it should be written in the patient's own words because the same words may mean different things to different people.

History of Present Illness (HPI)

This should be performed in a standard fashion. The questions are asked following the lead of the chief complaint. These questions should help you diagnose the pathological, anatomical, and/or physiological basis of your patient's complaint.

Many of your patients in the United States will be able to tell you what diseases they have suffered from in the past. The easy availability of old patient charts also gives you access to the specific details of your patient's medical and surgical history. Because of all this, many people start off the history as follows: "This is a 60-year-old white female, with a known case of hypertension, diabetes, trigeminal neuralgia. . . ." However, I think you should include only those elements of the past history that have a direct bearing on the present problem. For example, it is important to say that a patient is known to be HIV positive if he or she now presents with a cough. The rest of the past medical history should be described later under the "past medical history" heading.

Review of Systems (ROS)

During the ROS, you systematically ask the patient about symptoms attributable to each system. The list is usually written in the following order: general; skin; HEENT (head, eye, ear, nose, throat); neck; chest, including breast and respiratory system; cardiovascular, including heart and peripheral vascular system; abdomen, including genitalia; nervous system; hematological; endocrine; and psychiatric. You should ask about symptoms attributable to each system in a step-by-step fashion, looking at the positives and negatives that are relevant to the given case. This list should reflect your analytical thought process.

Past Medical and Surgical History

As noted above, it may be easier to obtain this history in the United States than in some other countries.

Social History

Tobacco Use You should ask about tobacco use in any form, (e.g., cigarettes, cigars, pipe, chewing, or snuff). In the case of cigarette smoking, give the pack-years. This is calculated as the number of (20-cigarette) packs smoked per day, multiplied by the number of years the person has smoked.

Alcohol Intake Alcoholism is underreported as well as underestimated by patients. This is where a thorough history can be very important. Several different screening questionnaires are available. The most popular one is the CAGE questionnaire (Am J Med 82:231,1987):

C—Ask if the patient felt that he or she should **c**ut down on alcohol intake.
A—Ask if the patient ever got ***a***nnoyed at somebody talking about his or her alcoholism.
G—Ask if the patient ever felt **g**uilty about his or her alcohol intake.
E—Ask if the patient ever needed alcohol as an ***e***ye-opener in the morning.

A "yes" answer to two or more questions has a 66 percent positive predictive value for alcohol abuse.

You should also ask about other forms of substance abuse. In the case of drug abuse, you should ask if the person snorts (sniffs), shoots (IV use), or ingests the drug.

Sexual Practices You should ask if the patient is sexually active. If yes, ask if the patient has sex with persons of the opposite, the same, or both sexes. Different sexual practices can predispose individuals to different types of diseases. Also inquire about the marital status of the patient. These questions should be asked of every patient.

Social Support System If the patient does not have an adequate support system at home, you should seek the help of a social worker in determining what you and the team can do to assist the patient.

Domestic Abuse You should always keep your eyes open for any clues to domestic abuse in your patients. The statistics show that victims underreport this problem. You should suspect domestic abuse in the following situations:

- When the type of injury is inconsistent with the history of the alleged cause of injury.
- When there is a past history of similar injuries.
- When there is a delay in seeking treatment for trauma.
- When the patient has a family member with a history of drug abuse.

Preventive and Screening History

I think this should be a feature of every good H&P. IMGs should be especially aware of preventive measures appropriate to the needs of American patients. The following areas should be emphasized:

- Counseling about safe sex practices
- Counseling about the importance of good diet and exercise
- Counseling about the benefits of quitting smoking; I personally feel that smoking should be listed as a disease in the history
- Rehabilitation options for patients with a history of alcohol or other substance abuse
- You should always be sensitive to the subtle signs of domestic violence. If detected, you should take the time to talk to the patient and ensure his or her safety.

Screening Measures It is recommended that patients in different age groups undergo certain laboratory tests or clinical examinations at specified intervals. These measures are recommended for early detection of several treatable diseases. The U.S. Preventive Services Task Force (USPSTF) is a government agency that develops recommendations for screening procedures. Other agencies that publish recommendations include the Canadian Task Force and the American College of Physicians (ACP). There is a wealth of information available on the

TABLE 12–1. Recommended Health Screening Measures

Blood pressure should be checked for the first time in any patient 18 years of age or older. The follow-up interval suggested is every 2 to 5 years, according to different authorities.

Clinical breast exam According to different authorities, this should be performed every 1 to 2 years in patients 50 to 69 years of age. The ACP recommends a first exam for all female patients 40+ years of age.

Pap smear is recommended every 3 years in women 18 to 65 or 20 to 65 or 18 to 69 years of age (different ranges are recommended by different authorities).

Stool for occult blood be tested annually for all patients 50+ years of age.

Sigmoidoscopy for early detection of colon cancer should be offered to every patient 50+ years of age. The USPSTF has not specified the frequency of testing for lack of evidence.

Mammography should be performed every 1 to 2 years in female patients 50 to 69 years of age.

Cholesterol should be tested in male patients between 35 and 65 years of age and in female patients between 45 and 65 years of age. The USPSTF recommends that the test be repeated every 5 years. The ACP leaves the frequency of this test up to the physician.

Internet. At *http://odphp.osophs.dhhs.gov*, you will find a detailed discussion about various screening measures. Different agencies sometimes differ on recommendations for a particular screening modality. This site gives the views of all the major agencies.

You should be familiar with the screening tests listed in Table 12–1. If your patient has high probability of developing a disease, for example, because of a family history of the disease, the screening test may need to be performed more often than is generally recommended, or additional tests may need to be performed.

Vaccines

Influenza vaccine should be offered each year to all patients 65 years of age, or older. It should also be offered to younger people who may come in contact with a high-risk population. This is done to prevent the transmission of the virus to high-risk groups. Other groups of patients who should be offered the vaccine include:

- Nursing home residents
- Children and adults with chronic cardiopulmonary disease
- Children and teenagers on chronic aspirin therapy
- Patients with diabetes, renal disease, hemoglobinopathy, and those receiving immunosuppressive therapy
- Women who are expected to be in second or third trimester of pregnancy during flu season

Pneumococcal vaccine should be offered to all patients over the age of 65 years. It is recommended for patients with asplenic sickle cell disease, as well as those patients with the following conditions:

- Cardiopulmonary disease
- Alcoholism
- Cirrhosis
- Cerebrospinal fluid leak
- Hodgkin's disease
- Chronic renal failure
- Lymphoma
- Chronic lymphocytic leukemia
- Multiple myeloma
- Nephrotic syndrome
- Organ transplant recipients
- HIV patients
- Patients receiving immunosuppressive therapy

A single dose is expected to give life-long immunity: However, revaccination is recommended for patients at very high risk of developing severe pneumococcal infection. These patients may include all of those with the conditions listed above.

TIPS FOR EFFECTIVE HISTORY-TAKING

Table 12–2 offers four tips to help IMGs improve the effectiveness of their history-taking technique.

TABLE 12–2. Four Tips for Effective History-Taking

1. Your patient should always feel that he or she has your undivided attention. Always sit in a relaxed posture while interviewing the patient and show genuine interest in what the patient has to say. The patient is always taking cues from your attitude. A good interviewer can extract much more information in a shorter time.
2. Always be professional in demeanor during your interaction with patients. Avoid false laughter and phony smiles. Do not talk down to your patients or sit in judgment of them. Evaluate them as other human beings with the help of the expertise provided by your medical training.
3. It is always easier to understand a person with an accent when he or she speaks slowly. It is especially important to speak slowly and clearly to your older hearing-impaired patients.
4. Do not become angry if you sense that a patient thinks you are less competent just because you are an IMG with an accent. The best way to change his or her mind is to provide excellent service.

PHYSICAL EXAMINATION

This is one of the areas where IMGs are likely to do better than U.S. medical graduates. The problem is that a significant number of IMGs who come to the United States are of the opinion that every patient in the United States gets a million-dollar workup. This leads them to downplay the importance of the H&P. However, a good history and thorough physical examination are indispensable parts of the practice of medicine anywhere in the world. As if to help me stress this point, the American Board of Internal Medicine (ABIM) has decided to include items on the board exams that will require examinees to have a good knowledge of physical exam techniques.

If you are one of those who has acquired good physical exam skills, stick to this systematic way of performing the exam. If you have not yet mastered these skills, learn them. I recommend that you cultivate the habit of carrying out a thorough examination on every patient. If you stick to this thorough routine, you will surprise yourself with your ability to home in on the diagnosis, more often than not.

They say "the eyes don't see what the mind does not know." But a systematic exam can reveal many findings whose relevance you may not know. Do not try sweeping them under the carpet. Instead, seek the significance for these findings. If you still cannot explain them, file them away in your brain data bank. Often you will find many of the answers over the next weeks, months, or years as you continue to read more.

This part of the chapter is in no way meant to be an exhaustive description of a complete physical examination. I presume you have read a good book on physical examination and that you know the systematic way of examining all systems. (One of the more popular books in the United States is Bates B, Bickley L, Hoekelman R: *A guide to physical examination and history taking*, 6th ed. Philadelphia: JP Lippincott, 1995.) Three points are worth stressing here, however:

1. Always follow a systematic approach when examining any system. The sequence (except in abdominal examination) should proceed the old-fashioned way; that is, inspection, palpation, percussion, and auscultation.

2. Develop a method of examining each system. Do it the same way on every patient you see. After a while, it will become a "two-minute affair" to do the complete exam. As an example, I have seen some doctors who always examine the abdomen in a clockwise fashion, starting with the liver, going in a circle, and ending in the middle of the abdomen. You may have to deviate from this routine once in a while. For instance, if a patient's most tender spot is over the liver, you should start examining on the left side.
3. Learn how to do each part of the exam the right way: First, because it is the right way; and second, because the exam done in the right way is supposed to be the most specific and sensitive for the diagnosis you are trying to make.

GENERAL EVALUATION

Start the physical examination with a statement indicating whether the patient is alert, awake, and oriented to time, place, and person. (AAOx3 is the common abbreviation for this.) State whether the patient was lying down, walking down the hall, or was sitting in a chair chatting with relatives when you saw the patient. This gives you, as well as others who read your note, a rough idea about the state of the patient at the time of your examination. This can become an important one-line reference in situations where a patient's condition later changes. You should state who gave the history and if you think the history is reliable. Do not refer to your patients as "crazy" just because they are doing something that is not part of your beliefs. Do not describe them as "difficult" because they are asking a question you do not have the answer to.

You can make a habit of putting certain other observations under this heading. These are the ones that you may feel do not fit into any of the other designated systems. For example, it is a good idea to describe any abnormalities of the skin here. This could also be a place to mention lymphadenopathy in different areas. You can write down any other observation that may be relevant to a given case here, as well.

VITAL SIGNS

A nurse or nursing assistant will usually record the vital signs. Make it a habit to check them yourself at least for situations in which the numbers do not seem to correlate with the clinical scenario. It is very important to understand the importance of accurate vital sign recording, especially in view of the fact that nursing assistants are not well trained to evaluate the clinical relevance of this data.

Blood Pressure (BP)

- The apparatus should always be reliable and the cuff size should be appropriate for the patient's size.
- If you suspect dissection of the aorta or peripheral vascular disease, check the BP in all four extremities.
- For patients in whom hypovolemia or autonomic dysfunction is suspected, check for orthostasis by assessing BP and pulse while the patient is lying down and again while standing.
- You can also look for paradoxical pulse if clinically indicated.

Pulse

- Make a habit of comparing the radial pulses by palpating both sides at the same time. You should also make a habit of comparing the radial to the femoral pulse. Other peripheral pulses such as the dorsalis pedis and posterior tibial may need to be palpated if you suspect peripheral vascular disease.
- Always take the pulse rate yourself. Note the rhythm and volume of the pulse.
- Different characteristics of pulses are well explained in most clinical examination books; for example, a slowly rising carotid pulse in severe aortic stenosis, a water hammer pulse in aortic regurgitation, and many more. You should try to get the feel of these particular characteristics as you assess patients with these diseases.

Respiratory Rate

The respiratory rate should always be counted when the patient is not aware that you are doing it.

Temperature

If the patient's temperature is too high or too low, you should insist on a rectal temperature.

Other Information

Other things that may be written in the same place as vital signs (when needed) are:

- Pulse oximetry (easily obtained by having the patient wear a probe on the finger) in patients with respiratory distress.
- Ventilator settings with special reference to the ventilator mode, set rate, patient's rate, tidal volume, positive end-expiratory pressure (PEEP), pressure support, and Fio_2.
- If the patient has a pulmonary artery (PA) catheter, you should write the latest numbers namely, central venous pressure (CVP), PA pressure, pulmonary capillary wedge pressure (PCWP), cardiac output and index, systemic vascular resistance (SVR), and pulmonary vascular resistance (PVR).

HEENT

The next area after vital signs is the examination of HEENT (***h***ead, ***e***ye, ***e***ar, ***n***ose, and ***t***hroat). Two common abbreviations used in this segment are PERRLA (pupils equal round and reactive to light and accommodation) and EOMI (extraoccular movements intact). It is easy to get into the habit of putting these abbreviations on every patient's chart without doing the required examination. However, you should *never* write up an exam that you have not done.

NECK

Look for the jugular venous pressure (JVP) with the patient in the proper position and the light from your penlight thrown tangentially across the neck. Check for any other abnormalities by going through the steps of inspection, palpation, percussion, and auscultation. You should palpate for the thyroid from behind with the patient's neck in a flexed and relaxed position.

CHEST

The chest consists of the front and back, including the breasts. If permitted by the patient, always expose the chest fully for examination.

Inspection

When looking for movement of the chest wall during breathing as well as comparing the movements on the two sides, bend down to bring your eyes to the level of the patient's chest. This can best be done by going to the foot end of the patient's bed with the patient lying supine.

Palpation

- Palpation of the breast should include palpation with the palmar aspect of the fingers as well as palpation between the fingers. You should also gently squeeze the nipple to check for any discharge.
- To check for vocal fremitus, ask the patient to say repeatedly "1, 2, 3." As the patient does so, you should feel the resonance of the sound waves through the intercostal spaces with the ulnar aspect of your palm. Always compare both sides of the same area. For example after palpating in the right infraclavicular area, go to the left infraclavicular, and then to the right mammary area, followed by the left mammary area, and so on.
- During palpation, always check for the position of the trachea.

Percussion

When examining the chest, heavy percussion is used. Here again, you should compare both sides as described above. This makes it easier to appreciate any differences between the two sides. Percussion of the chest is also used to demarcate the upper level of liver dullness.

Auscultation

Auscultation of the chest should be performed with special reference to the character and intensity of breath sounds and any accompaniments, namely crackles, ronchi, or pleural rub. You should also assess vocal resonance (the auscultatory counterpart of vocal fremitus) and whispering pectoriloquy if need be. Compare both sides in the same area in quick succession. You should auscultate three areas on each side of the front, namely, infraclavicular area, mammary area, and inframammary area. You should also examine the axillary and infraaxillary areas on each side. On the back, auscultate the suprascapular, scapular, and infrascapular areas on each side. This routine helps you probe all major areas of each lung.

Do not auscultate too close to the spine, especially in the higher thoracic area, as the normal character of breathing can be bronchial here. This can confuse you into making a diagnosis of a cavity or consolidation.

HEART

Inspection

You should look for any pulsation over the chest. Observe for the point of maximal impulse (PMI).

Palpation

This segment should start with an honest attempt to locate the PMI. You may not succeed all the time. After you find the PMI, try to classify the apex beat as being of a tapping or heaving type. This palpation should be performed with the palmar aspect of the distal phalanx of your finger.

The heaving type of apex pulse is the one that slowly lifts your finger with each stroke, something like a slow-rising wave. This should be followed by palpation for any thrill. In the cardiac exam, you should make a habit of doing each part of the exam in all valve areas in sequence. I like to start at the apex (mitral area), then sweep over to the lower end of left sternum (tricuspid area), then go along the left side of the sternum, up to the second left intercostal space (pulmonary area), and finish with the second right intercostal space (aortic area). Some people refer to the second right intercostal area as the A1 area and the area to the left of the sternum as the A2 area because an aortic insufficiency (AI) murmur is best heard in the latter area.

Palpation of these areas should be followed by palpation of the left parasternal area for the heave. This should be done by keeping the base of the palmar aspect of your hand along the left parasternal area. Your wrist crease should be oriented along the length of the patient. You should feel for any lift of the hand. For a subtle heave, you should bring your eyes to the level of the patient's chest and *look* for any lift.

Percussion

In this era of easily available echocardiograms and X-rays, I do not feel there is any utility in doing percussion to delineate the cardiac border. The argument in favor of doing this evaluation (which has low accuracy at best) is that there could still be situations where these diagnostic tools are unavailable. However, I would still argue that this exam is not sufficiently reliable to open someone's chest or stick a needle in this area purely on the basis of your percussion of the cardiac border.

Auscultation

You should make a habit of auscultating all the areas in sequence, as explained above. This segment of the exam should always include auscultation of the carotids. Auscultation of the heart is always a scary proposition for new medical students. In contrast to the examination of the lungs, where they can ask the patient to breathe at different rates, here, they are confronted with an organ that they cannot slow down in order to better analyze their various findings. For a new examiner, it is a feeling of trying to count the passengers sitting in a moving train as it whizzes by.

Following are several problems relating to auscultation of the heart that I have identified over several years of working with physicians at different levels of training:

- The identification of S1 and S2 (first heart sound and second heart sound, respectively) should be the first step during the auscultation. It may be difficult sometimes to identify which sound is S1 and which one is S2. Here is a tip: Perform the palpation of carotids simultaneously with auscultation. The sound heard while the carotid upstroke hits your finger is S1. This tip can take away a lot of your anxiety. Once you have identified S1, it is easy to figure out that anything between S1 and S2 is systolic in timing and that anything between S2 and the next S1 is diastolic.
- Next focus your attention on the character and intensity of these two sounds.
- This done, you can now easily appreciate any extraneous sound, if present. Beyond that you have to set out trying to find various characteristics of the extraneous sound(s) in order to be able to know its/their significance.
- Always be aware of the correct patient position and the part of the stethoscope (bell or diaphragm) to be used when listening for a sound. Examples include left lateral position for mitral stenosis (MS) murmur, and patient sitting up and bending forward with breath held in expiration for an AI murmur.

- Also, be aware of the dynamic auscultation. This can markedly increase the yield of your exam. As an example, a hand squeeze may make a faint MS murmur prominent.
- You should be aware of characteristics of different sounds. This can help in diagnosis and differential diagnosis. For example, a pansystolic murmur heard in the area around the tricuspid and mitral area that increases in intensity on deep inspiration is likely to be a tricuspid regurgitation (TR) murmur rather than a mitral regurgitation (MR) murmur.
- One thing that helps the more experienced practitioners to perform auscultation more effectively is that they know what to expect even before beginning to auscultate. The flip side is that some people like to claim that they can hear extra sounds that nobody else can hear. As an example, some people may get an ego trip out of saying that they hear an S3 (without actually being able to appreciate it) in all the patients with left ventricular dysfunction.
- Finally in my experience, an honest and thorough clinical exam can often guide you correctly when the high-tech machines give you an occasional wrong result.

Other Areas

Even a limited cardiac exam should always end with an examination of other systems that are relevant to the given case. Examples might include:

- Looking for signs of Marfan's syndrome in a patient with AI. Similarly, perform a brief exam to look for any signs that could possibly help you make the diagnosis or quantify the severity of a given cardiac disease.
- Assessing for other congenital abnormalities in a patient with congenital heart disease.
- Looking for extracardiac signs of infective endocarditis.

ABDOMEN AND SPINE

Remember that the abdominal exam consists of four parts: (1) the abdomen proper, (2) the back and spine, (3) the genitalia, and (4) the rectal exam. You should be familiar with the abbreviations used to report findings for this system in U.S. hospitals. These are not internationally recognized abbreviations, and I am not trying to prompt their use as such. I am including them here simply to prevent you from becoming confused when you see them during the initial stages of your training in the United States.

N/V/D—nausea/vomiting/diarrhea
BRBPR—bright red blood per rectum
T/R/G—tenderness/rebound/guarding

My suggestions for ensuring a proper examination of this system follow.

- The sequence followed in the abdominal examination should be (1) inspection, (2) auscultation, (3) percussion, and (4) palpation. *This is different from the sequence followed for other systems.*
- Always warn the patient before beginning the abdominal exam. Your hands as well as the stethoscope should be at a comfortable temperature. Your palpation should be gentle. If a patient has a tender area, always start away from that area and slowly and gently advance toward the tender spot.
- An experienced person performing an abdominal exam should look like an artist working on a canvas with the soft sweeps of a paint brush. Conversely, the wrong technique can look crude and cruel to the patient as well as to anyone else watching the process of the examination.
- You should know the proper method of palpating for different abdominal organs. You should also know the characteristics of different masses; namely, location, movement with respiration, and so forth. This can help you greatly in making a diagnosis. It can be helpful to draw a simple diagram depicting how the mass feels to you.
- Never underestimate the significance of tenderness, guarding, or rebound in an abdominal exam.
- Always finish the exam of the front of the abdomen with an examination of hernia sites. Then you can go to the back. The examination of the genitalia is more conveniently performed just prior to the rectal examination.
- Percussion in the abdominal exam should always be soft. This means soft taps. You should have your ears close to the abdomen to be able to appreciate any subtle difference.
- Auscultation of abdomen is another important step. You should be aware that the frequency of bowel sounds could be as low as once every 30 minutes. Apart from bowel sounds, you should also assess for abdominal bruit.
- You can never go wrong by performing a rectal exam on every patient. At the end of the rectal exam, you should do a Guaic test on the stool sample on your gloved finger. This test detects occult blood in stools. In the United States, small pads are available; you can apply the stool sample to the suggested site, apply some liquid developer, and read the result within a few minutes.

CENTRAL NERVOUS SYSTEM (CNS) EXAMINATION

A thorough CNS exam can be very time consuming. The CNS exam should include the components listed in Table 12–3 and described on the following pages.

Higher Functions

This segment of the exam should include:

- The patient's ability to speak and understand speech
- Evaluation of reading and writing ability appropriate to the patient's educational background
- A quick mini mental status examination

Cranial Nerves

This portion of the exam can be completed in a few minutes if you pick a routine and stick to it. The following routine is suggested for assessing the cranial nerves (CNs):

- CN1 (olfactory nerve) assessment can be omitted in an everyday exam in the absence of symptoms referable to this nerve.
- CN2 assessment should include a rough assessment of visual acuity, light reflex (direct and consensual), fundus exam, and bedside peripheral field by confrontation method. Visual acuity can be roughly checked by asking the patient to identify any object or figure from several feet away. If the patient cannot do so, ask him or her to count how many of your fingers you hold up at different distances. Failing that, you should use your pen-

TABLE 12–3. Components of the Central Nervous System Examination

Higher functions
Cranial nerves
Motor system
Sensory system
Cerebellum
Gait

light to check the light perception of each eye. The confrontation test is performed as follows: Seating yourself face to face with the patient with your eyes at the same level as those of the patient. To check the left eye, ask the patient to close his or her right eye and then close your left eye (i.e., the eyes facing each other should be open). Now, ask the patient to look into your eyes and not move the eye. Position your fingers in all quadrants on both sides and ask the patient to count your fingers. Repeat the same procedure with the other eye. Remember, this is a comparison of the patient's peripheral field with that of the examiner, assuming that the examiner has a normal peripheral field. Thus, the examiner, too, should look straight into the patient's eyes and should be able to see the fingers that he or she expects the patient to see.

- CNS 3, 4, and 6 should be checked by evaluating the movements of the eyeball. CN 3 is additionally responsible for consensual reflex to light. Ptosis can appear with CN 3 or sympathetic nerve involvement.
- CN 5 should be checked by evaluating the sensations on the face and the corneal reflex. The motor part can be checked by asking the patient to clench the teeth and then feeling for temple and jaw muscle.
- CN 7 should be checked by evaluating the patient's ability to do the following:
    (1) Wrinkle the forehead while sitting by attempting to look straight toward the ceiling without extending the neck.
    (2) Close the eyes by screwing them tight.
    (3) Also ask the patient to give you a big smile to check for symmetry of the nasolabial folds. (The request to "show me your teeth" in an attempt to assess this area will occasionally generate the answer "I do not have any teeth.") If findings are abnormal, you should determine whether the facial nerve palsy involves the forehead and eyelids (infranuclear facial palsy) or not (supranuclear).
- CN 8 can be crudely checked using the whisper test.
- CN 9 and 10 can be checked by asking the patient to say "ah". Watch for the symmetrical rise of the soft palate. The gag reflex is another function of these nerves. Evaluation of this reflex can be an unpleasant experience for many patients. A badly performed gag reflex test can make an enemy out of your patient. If

the gag reflex is absent, curb your tendency to be more vigorous in an effort to "extract" the reflex from the patient. Some normal patients may have an absent gag reflex.

- CN 11 can be checked by asking the patient to shrug and move the neck sideways against resistance.
- CN 12 can be checked by asking the patient to stick out the tongue and looking for any deviation to either side. Also look for any tongue atrophy or fasciculations.

Motor System

This portion of the exam should include the following components:

- Inspection: For any abnormal movements, atrophy, or fasciculations.
- Muscle tone: Check the tone by passively moving various joints of the upper and lower extremities.
- Power: Evaluate the power in view of the patient's overall condition and compare the two sides of the patient. When you are asking the patient to squeeze your fingers, offer only two fingers, neither of which should have a ring on it. Always grade the power from 1 to 5.
- Reflexes: These should include the biceps, brachioradial, abdominal, knee, and ankle reflexes. Always compare the two sides. The abdominal reflex may be absent in normal patients. Cremasteric and anal reflexes can be useful in localizing the spinal or root lesions in some situations, but these do not need to be evaluated as a part of the everyday exam. The exam should conclude with assessment of the plantar reflex.

Sensory System

This portion of the exam should evaluate:

- Pain sensation with a pin. Always compare the two sides in the same area.
- Touch sensation with cotton.
- Position and vibration: Many older patients have impaired vibration sense.
- Cortical sensation: Inscribe a numeral from 1 to 9 on the patient's hand or plantar aspect of the foot using a blunt object.

The patient should be able to tell you the number without seeing you do it. Cortical sensations should be checked only if other sensations are normal.

Cerebellum

Cerebellar function can be checked using the finger-to-nose and shin-heel test. You can also ask the patient to alternately supine and pronate, while observing for lag on either side. Cerebellar tests are not reliable in patients with significant pyramidal tract impairment.

Gait

The patient's gait can provide clues about pyramidal, cerebellar, or some (cerebral) lobar dysfunction. Before observing the patient walking, ask him or her to stand with the feet together and eyes closed. If the patient sways, this is a positive Romberg's sign, which is suggestive of posterior column involvement. You need to be very careful in interpreting this sign. The exact significance of the test is lost if the patient has motor weakness or cerebellar involvement.

LOWER EXTREMITIES

The lower extremities are examined next, after the completion of the CNS exam. It is abbreviated LE. This segment is where you would note the presence of edema, any color or temperature change, or dilated veins.

MUSCULOSKELETAL EXAMINATION

If the individual case demands, you may need to perform a musculoskeletal exam. This would include inspection, palpation, and assessment of range of motion (ROM) of different joints.

WRITING THE LABS ON THE CHART

After completing the write-up of the exam findings, the lab results are next entered. In the United States, the chemistry results are written in a unique grid pattern that can be very confusing to the ignorant. An example is provided in Figure 12–1.

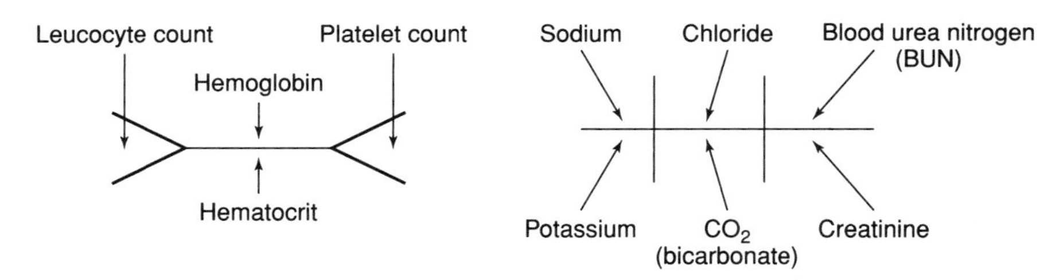

FIGURE 12–1. Grid format used in the U.S. for writing the chemistry results on a chart.

H&P AND DAILY PROGRESS NOTES

A detailed note on every new admission should have five components:

1. History
2. Physical examination
3. Relevant lab results
4. Assessment
5. Plan

The daily progress note should be written in the SOAP format, as follows:

Subjective
Objective
Assessment
Plan

S (SUBJECTIVE)

Under this head you should write the subjective feelings of the patient. These should be written verbatim as far as possible: "I couldn't sleep last night." "I haven't moved my bowels for 5 days," "When can I go home, doc? I've got a lot of things to take care of at home." You should give the pride of place to the patient's concerns in this section, even if you feel they have nothing to do with the admitting diagnosis. You should also put a lot of your effort toward taking care of your patient's complaints or concerns.

O (OBJECTIVE)

You should write down your physical examination findings here, followed by the lab results.

A (ASSESSMENT)

Under this heading, you should write what you think about the overall condition of the patient. This is the place where you can write what you think about the diagnosis and the rationale behind your decision. For example, suppose you have a patient with a complaint of tiredness and anemia. You can write, "I suspect hematological malignancy as the patient has marked splenomegaly and lymphadenopathy." You should discuss different problems under different heads. An example is shown below:

The daily progress notes should always be written in SOAP format.

- *Congestive heart failure (CHF):* Patient is know to have CHF. This episode may have been precipitated by atrial fibrillation. Feels better today as compared to yesterday.
- *Hypertension:* Well controlled. The patient says her BP has been around 120/70 on measurements at home.
- *High BUN:* Possibly due to aggressive diuresis.
- *Diabetes mellitus type 2:* Poorly controlled. Blood sugars have been between 250 and 350 during the hospital stay.

P (PLAN)

In this segment, you should write how you plan to deal with all the issues enumerated previously under the assessment. The plan can be in the form of medications, investigations, referrals, and so on. Continuing with the example given above, you might write the following:

- *CHF:* Will continue diuretics and ace inhibitors. Will decrease the dose of diuretics in view of satisfactory diuresis and rising BUN. Will start small-dose beta blockers and increase as tolerated.
- *Hypertension:* Will continue same medications.
- *Rising BUN:* Will watch for response to decreased dose of diuretics.
- *DM type 2:* Will call endocrinology consult for help with sugar control.

ELECTROCARDIOGRAPHY (ECG OR EKG)

In this part of the chapter, my goal is to help you become proficient in detecting the cardiac abnormalities that can be life threatening if undetected. Several electrocardiogram (ECG) tracings are included here only to familiarize you with specific findings. Keep in mind that an ECG alone in the absence of the history has little significance. The same ECG can be normal and abnormal in different clinical settings. At the residency level, I recommend that you err more on the side of over-calling the abnormalities. Discuss any abnormal-looking ECGs with your senior resident and let him or her make the decision about the seriousness of the situation. In this way, you can learn on a case-by-case basis without harming any of your patients.

Always compare the patient's ECG with a prior ECG, if available. The ECG technician may be able to help you find a previous ECG of the patient, if available. A new change has much more significance than an abnormality that has persisted for years.

First let us look at an ECG that is within normal limits (ECG 12–1). You should develop a method for reading every ECG. An easy five-step method is as follows:

1. Calculate the heart rate. Determine if the heart rate is within normal limits or if bradycardia or tachycardia is present.

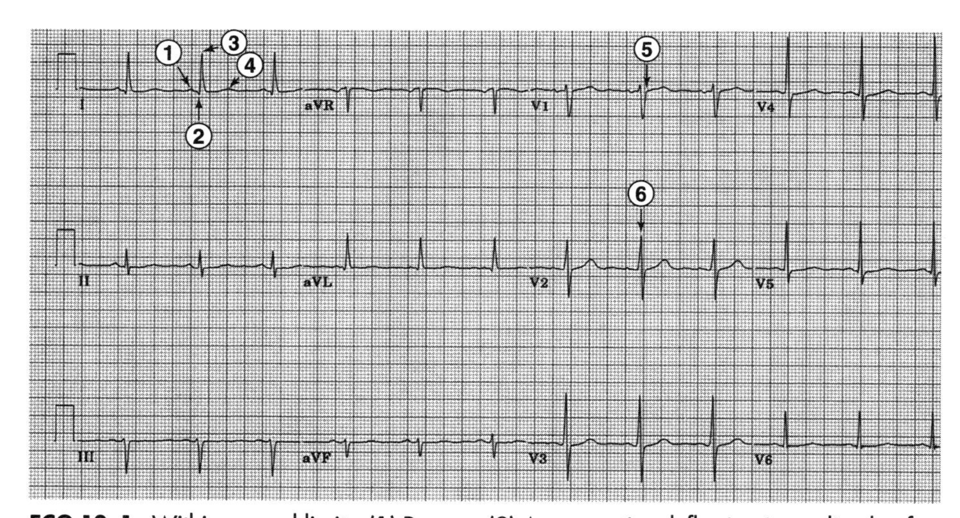

ECG 12–1. Within normal limits. (1) P wave. (2) Any negative deflection immediately after the P wave is called the Q wave. (3) First positive deflection immediately after the Q wave is the R wave. (4) The T wave is the deflection after the ST segment. (5) A negative deflection after the R wave is the S wave. (6) There may be leads with no Q wave; the positive deflection after the P wave here is the R wave. Take the time to review which leads represent which wall of the ventricle.

2. See if the rate is regular. If not, what is the pattern of irregularity?
3. Look at the size and shape of the P wave and the QRS complex. Focus on the relationship of the P and QRS complexes.
4. Measure the different intervals and see if they are within normal limits. Important intervals are the PR, QRS, and QT.
5. Look at the ST segment and the T waves.

Admittedly this is not a complete list of things to look for, but it provides a quick overview.

ISCHEMIA AND MYOCARDIAL INFARCTION (MI)

The diagnosis of these two conditions should start with a good history.

Ischemia

This condition is diagnosed from ST depression or T-wave inversion in the ECG. The ST depression can be one of three types:

1. Horizontal: This type of ST depression is highly suggestive of ischemia (ECG 12–2).
2. Upsloping: Whenever you see upsloping ST depression (see ECG 12–11), you should follow the ST segment to a point 0.08 seconds (2 small squares on the graph) after the J point. (This is a point where the S wave ends and the ST segment starts.)

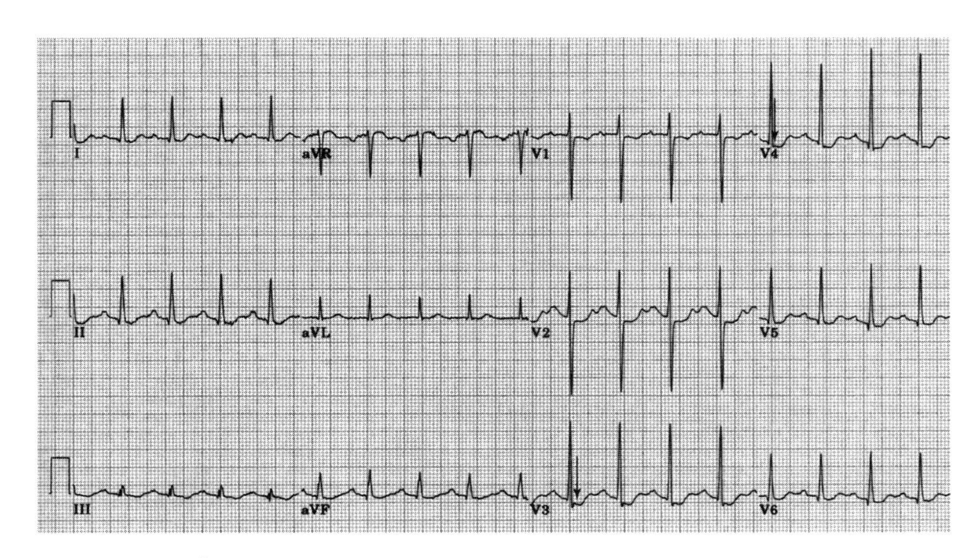

ECG 12–2. ST depression (*arrows*).

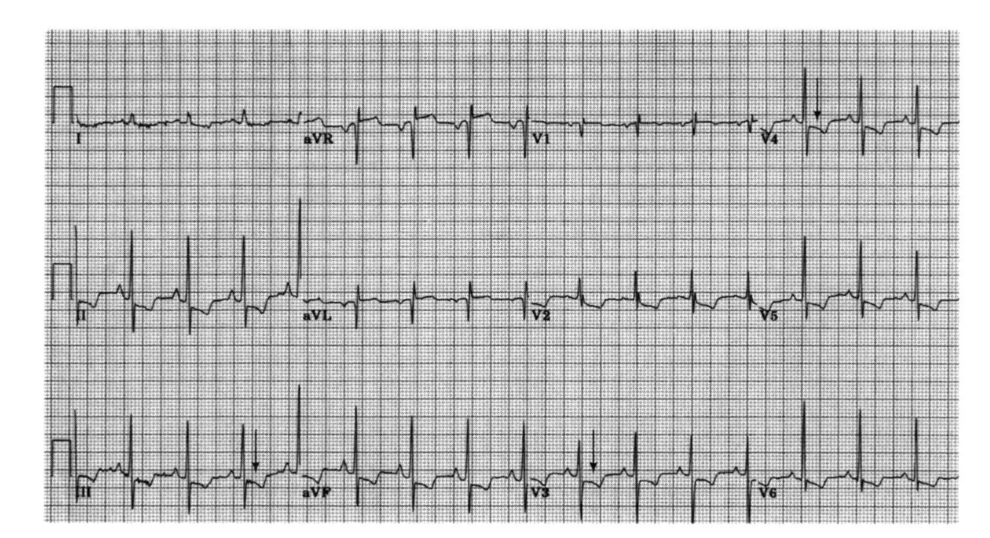

ECG 12–3. Downsloping ST depression (*arrows*).

Compare this point to the PR segment for calculation of ST depression. A 1- to 2-mm (1 mm = 1 small square) ST depression can be suggestive of ischemia in the right setting. Look at the leads showing this abnormality. If this change is found in all the leads and not in the leads corresponding to a particular vascular territory, it is more likely to be a nonspecific change.

3. Downsloping: This is seen in ECG 12–3. The method of analyzing this depression is the same as that followed for upsloping depression. This type of depression can also occur as part of a drug effect.

T-wave inversion can be a sign of ischemia. It is important to compare these findings with the patient's previous ECG. Changes that have persisted for years may have little new significance. An ST depression or T-wave inversion that is transient and keeps changing, especially when accompanied by the appropriate symptoms, is more suggestive of ischemia.

Acute MI

The nomenclature of acute MI follows two lines. One basis of classification is according to the wall represented by the ECG graph; for example, anterior wall MI or inferior wall MI. This classification has remained consistent over the years. The other basis for classification is an attempt to differentiate whether the patient has had an infarction of a part or of the whole thickness of the heart wall on the basis of ECG findings. Initially the terms subendocardial (for partial wall) and transmural (for full-wall thickness) infarction were used, with the distinction being made on the basis of the presence or absence of the Q wave. Later, the sensitivity and specificity of the Q wave for the diagnosis of the extent of heart wall involvement was thought to be less than desirable and the terms were changed to Q wave and non-Q wave infarction. More recently, the terms have been changed to "MI with ST elevation" and "MI without ST elevation" based simply on whether or not the patient with high cardiac enzymes had an ST elevation on presentation.

ST Elevation

Any ST elevation should prompt you to seek the help of your senior resident. An ST elevation that is not acute MI can indicate one of the following conditions:

- Benign early repolarization abnormality. Review of the patient's previous ECG is important here. If the patient had the same type of ST elevation on another ECG in the past while in the asymptomatic state, the change is more likely to be benign.
- Pericarditis. This condition will cause ST elevation in almost all the leads. The history will be different from that suggestive of MI.
- A dyskinetic segment. A patient who has had an MI may keep showing persistent ST elevation as a result of a dyskinetic segment in the area of the MI. However, you should be cautious about attributing these changes to a dyskinetic segment in a patient experiencing typical ischemic chest pain.

Once you see the ST elevation suggestive of acute MI (ECG 12–4), you should immediately initiate treatment. You should now direct your attention to the territory represented by the leads with ST elevation. As a quick review:

1. Leads II, III, and aVF represent the inferior wall.
    a. Whenever you see changes in the inferior wall, do the right-sided ECG. This can help in diagnosing right ventricular infarction, which frequently occurs in association with inferior wall infarction. This knowledge in turn alerts you to the fact that that patient can have severe hypotension in response to the administration of nitroglycerin. The treatment for a patient with hypotension and right ventricular infarction is intravenous fluid bolus. This is one of the rare cases in cardiology in which you give IV fluids to a cardiac

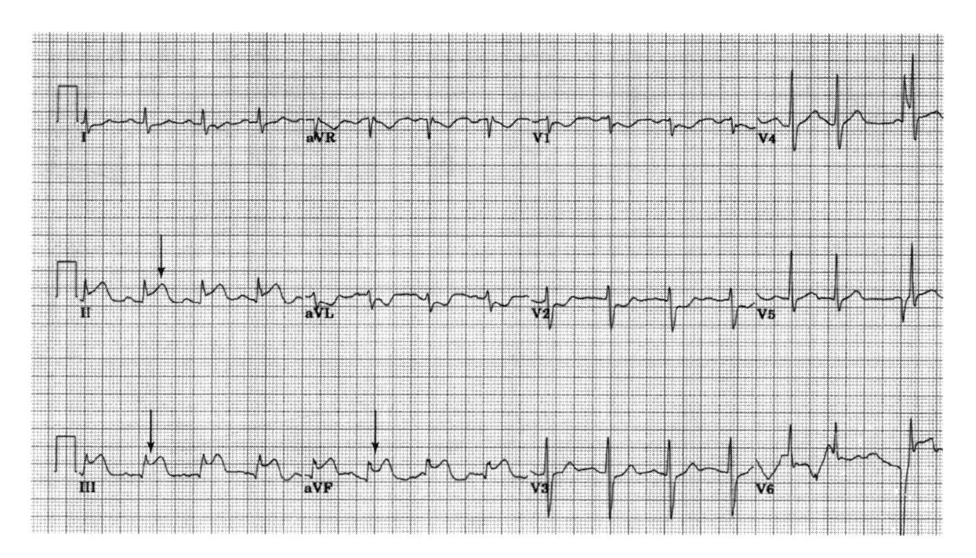

ECG 12–4. ST elevation in leads II, III, and aVF (*arrows*). Inferior wall MI.

patient. In other situations, most doctors are very wary of giving fluids to their patients with *any* heart problem (not necessarily rightly so).

b. You should next direct your attention to V1. A new, tall R wave with an upward T wave could be an indicator of posterior wall infarction.

2. Leads I, aVL, and/or V5–6 represent the lateral wall.
3. Leads V1–2 represent the septum.
4. Leads V3–4 represent the anterior wall.
5. Extensive anterior wall MI can cause ST changes in all precordial leads.

Bundle Branch Block

It is important to diagnose the bundle branch block because a newly appearing block could represent acute ischemia. Pulmonary embolism can cause acute right bundle branch block (RBBB). On the other hand, you may not see typical changes of ischemia or MI in patients who already have bundle branch block. The ECG of such patients may be so deformed that the ST–T changes may loose their usual specificity. It is very easy to diagnose bundle branch block:

1. First measure the QRS duration. If there is no Q wave (first negative deflection after P), start the measurement at the takeoff of the R wave. The ending point should be the end of the S wave. The suggested upper limit is 0.10 seconds, meaning

2½ small squares on the graph. If it is more than that, the diagnosis of intraventricular conduction defect is made.

2. Now focus your attention on V1 and V6. If there is an rSR pattern in V1 and a persistent and or slurred S wave in V6, the diagnosis is RBBB (ECG 12–5). If there is a broad R wave in V 6 and a broad S wave in V1, the diagnosis of left bundle branch block (LBBB) is made (ECG 12–6). As described previously, BBB also comes with ST–T changes.

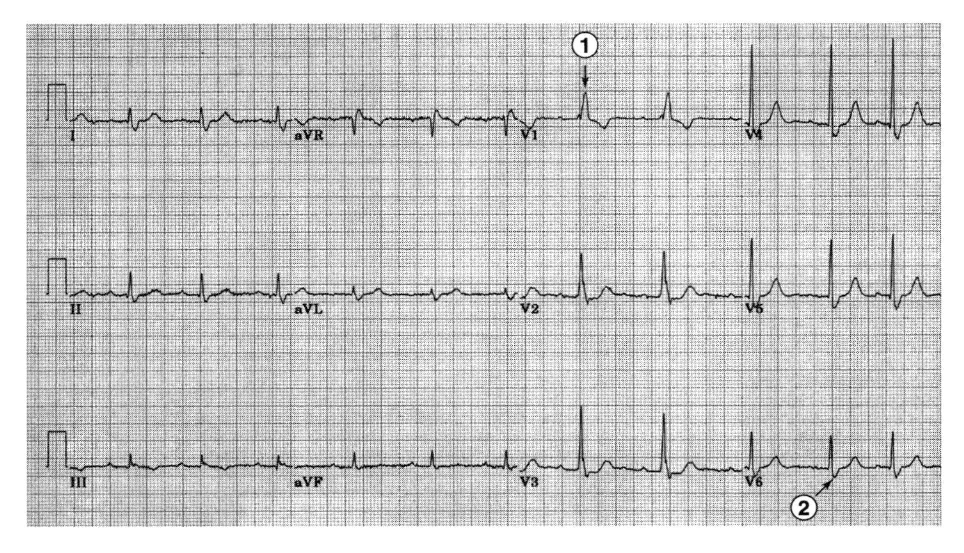

ECG 12–5. Right bundle branch block. Note the broad QRS, tall R wave in V1 (1), and slurred S wave in V6 (2).

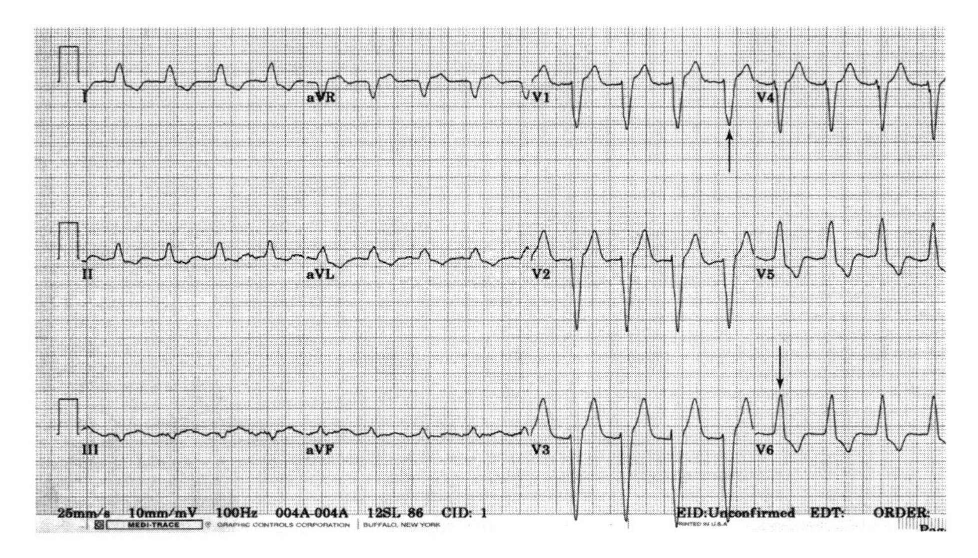

ECG 12–6. Left bundle branch block. Note the broad QRS complexes, deep S wave in V1, and tall R wave in V6 (*arrows*).

Diagnosing Ischemia or MI in the Presence of Bundle Branch Block

A complete history of symptoms is extremely important in this particular situation. If the patient has typical chest pain with no significant changes in the ECG, treat it like unstable angina until more data are available.

RBBB does not limit our ability to diagnose MI as much as LBBB does. The significance of the difficulty of diagnosis of MI in the presence of LBBB is reflected in numerous well-designed studies that have sought to improve our chances of diagnosis in this situation. In one of the largest studies published in the *New England Journal of Medicine* (Sgarbossa E, et al: Electrocardiographic diagnosis of evolving acute myocardial infarction in the presence of left bundle branch block. N Engl J Med 1996;334:481–487), the following findings were found to be useful:

- ST segment elevation ≥1 mm and concordant with the QRS complex (in the same direction as the main force of the QRS complex) had a sensitivity and specificity of 73% and 92%, respectively. (Refer to Chapter 13 for definitions of sensitivity and specificity.)
- ST depression ≥1 mm in lead V1, V2, or V3 had a sensitivity and specificity of 25% and 96%, respectively.
- ST elevation ≥5 mm and discordant with the ORS complex (when the main force of the QRS is negative) had a sensitivity and specificity of 31% and 92%, respectively.

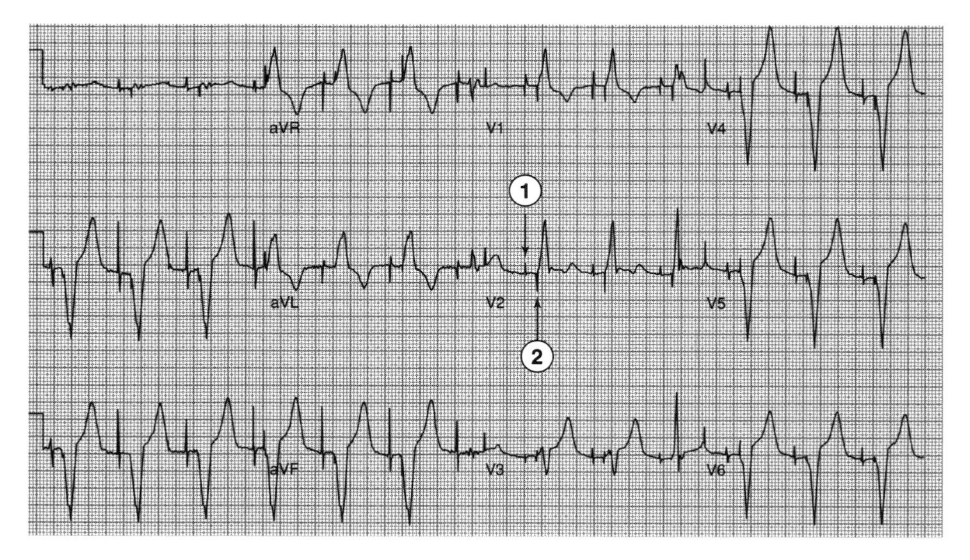

ECG 12–7. Dual chamber pacemaker rhythm. Note the pacing spike from the atrial lead followed by atrial depolarization (1), and the pacing spike from the ventricular lead followed by ventricular depolarization (2).

- A positive T wave in lead V5 or V6 had a sensitivity and specificity of 26% and 92%, respectively
- Left-axis deviation had a sensitivity and specificity of 72% and 48%, respectively.

PACED BEATS

You should be able to identify the rhythm created by a pacemaker as opposed to the patient's own rhythm (ECG 12–7).

ARRHYTHMIAS

It is very easy to diagnose arrhythmias if you use the algorithms shown in Figures 12–2 and 12–3. Look at ECGs 12–8 through 12–17 and try to make a diagnosis with the help of these algorithms.

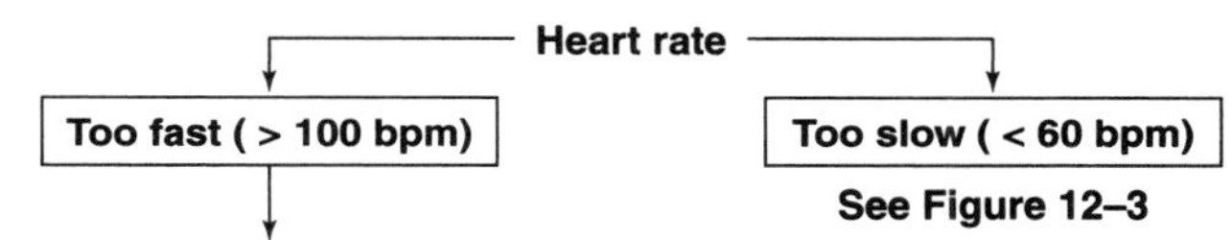

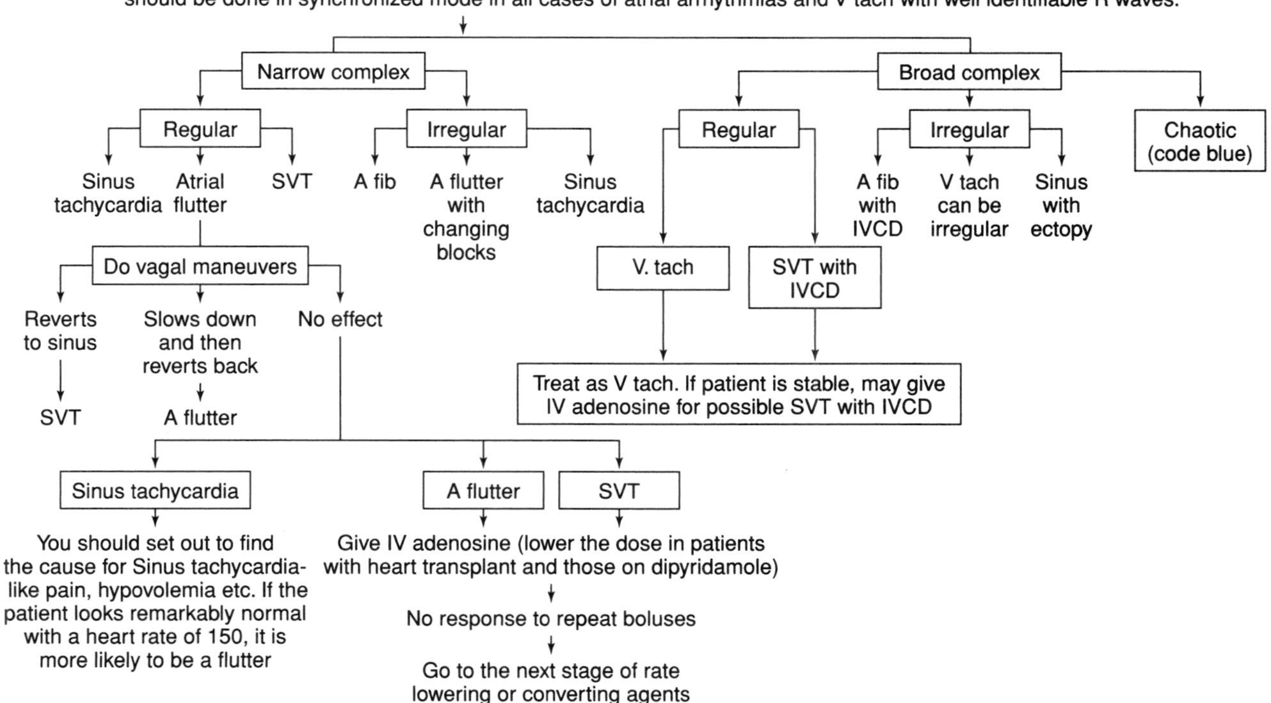

FIGURE 12–2. Algorithm for diagnosing an arrhythmia characterized by heart rate > 100 bpm. A fib, atrial fibrillation; BP, blood pressure; IVCD, intraventricular conduction defect; SVT, supraventricular tachycardia; V tach, ventricular tachycardia. Note that the ventricular rate in A fib may not always be more than 100 bpm.

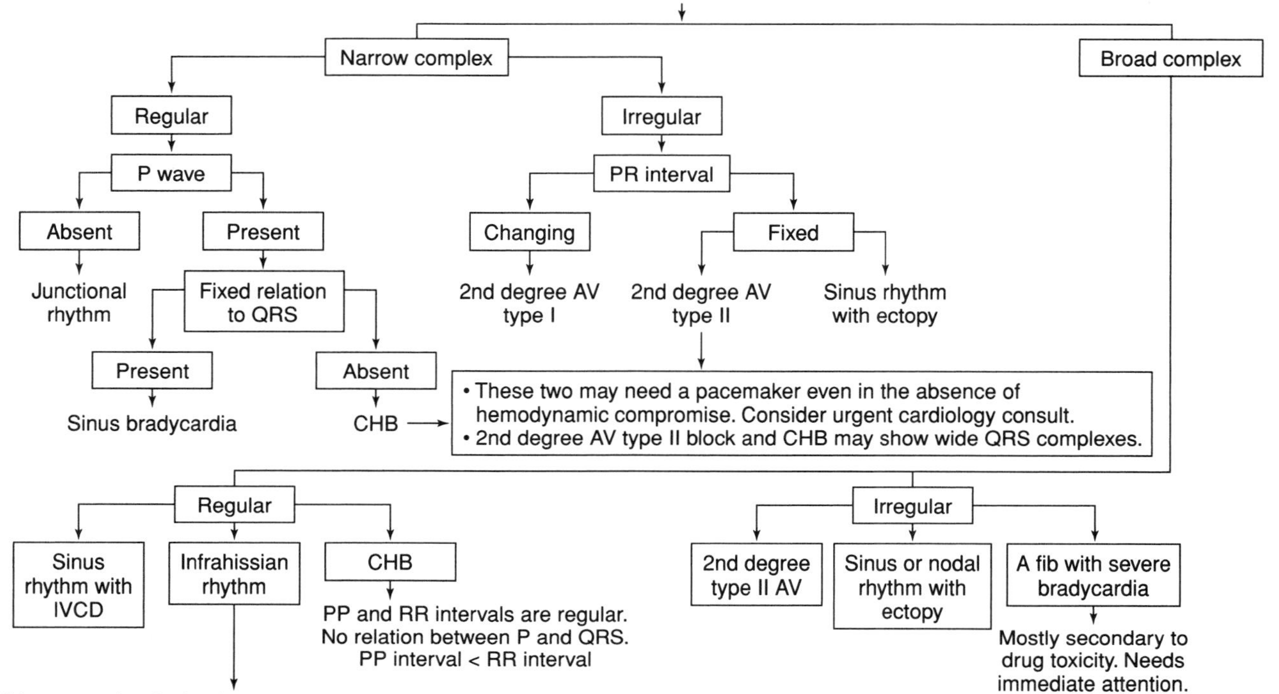

FIGURE 12–3. Algorithm for diagnosing an arrhythmia characterized by a heart rate < 60 bpm. A fib, atrial fibrillation; AV, atrioventricular block; CHB, complete heart block; IVCD, intraventricular conduction defect.

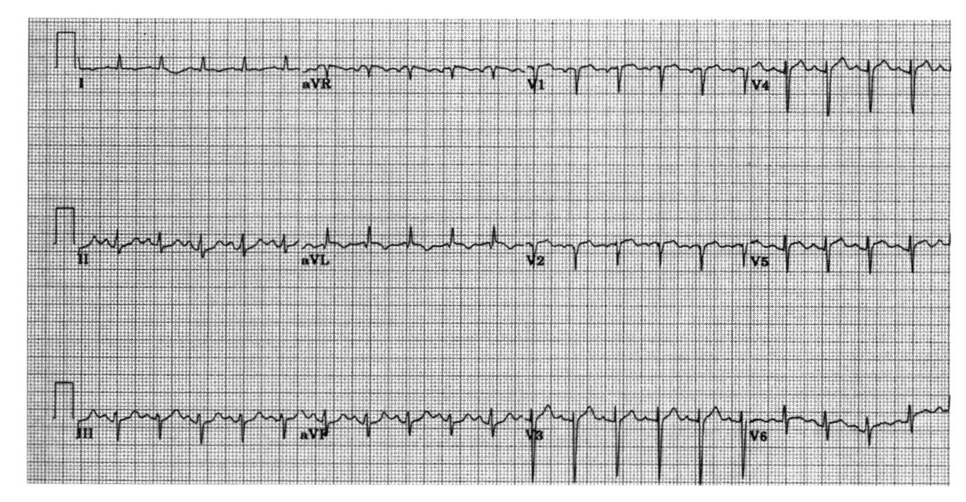

ECG 12–8. Sinus tachycardia. heart rate > 100 bpm.

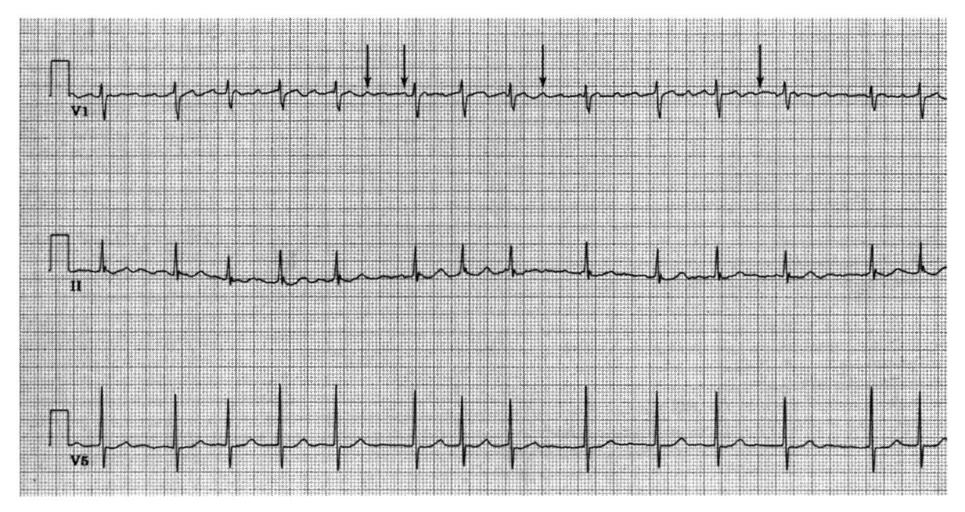

ECG 12–9. (Rhythm strip.) Atrial fibrillation. Note the deflections that may be confused with flutter waves (*arrows*); however, the flutter waves should maintain their shape in a single lead and should appear at a predictable interval (unlike this tracing).

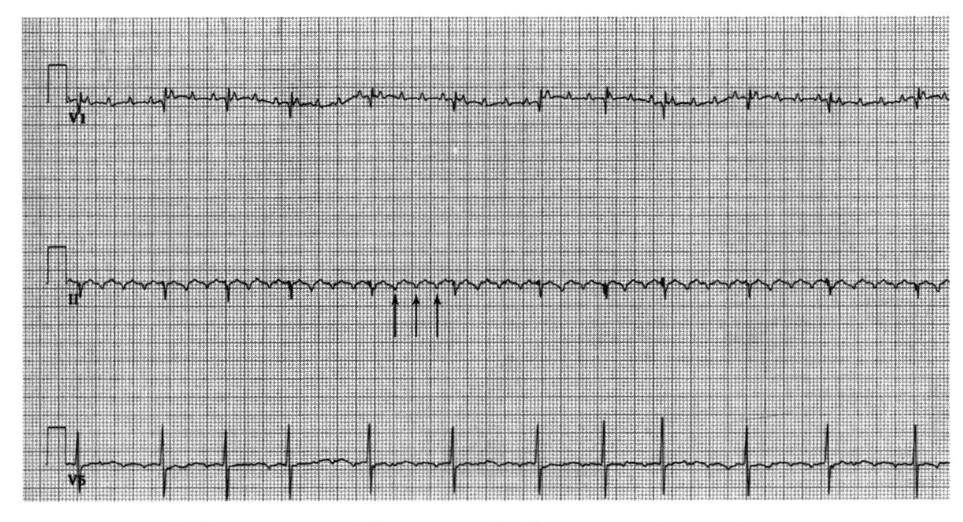

ECG 12–10. (Rhythm strip.) Atrial flutter. Note the flutter waves (*arrows*).

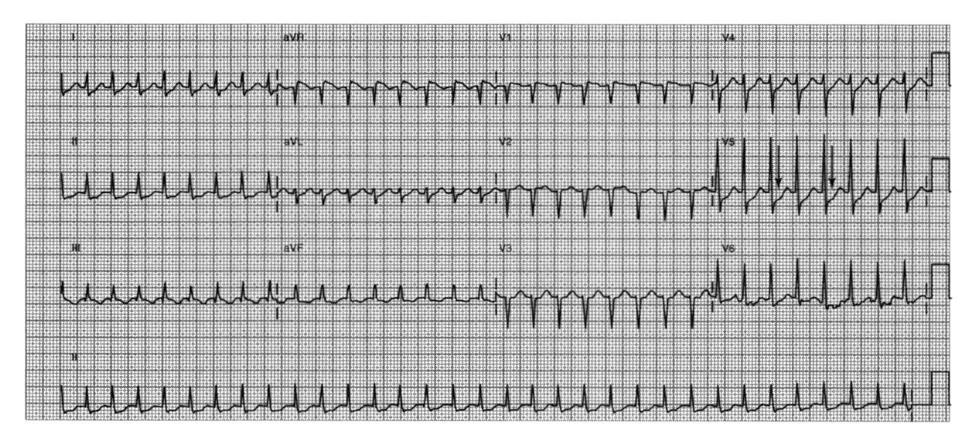

ECG 12–11. Supraventricular tachycardia. Also note the upsloping ST segment depression (*arrow*).

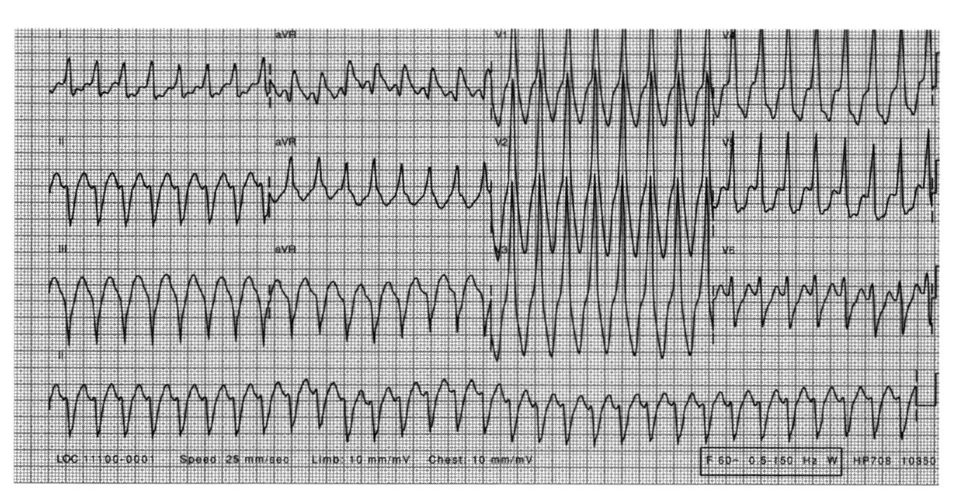

ECG 12–12. Ventricular tachycardia.

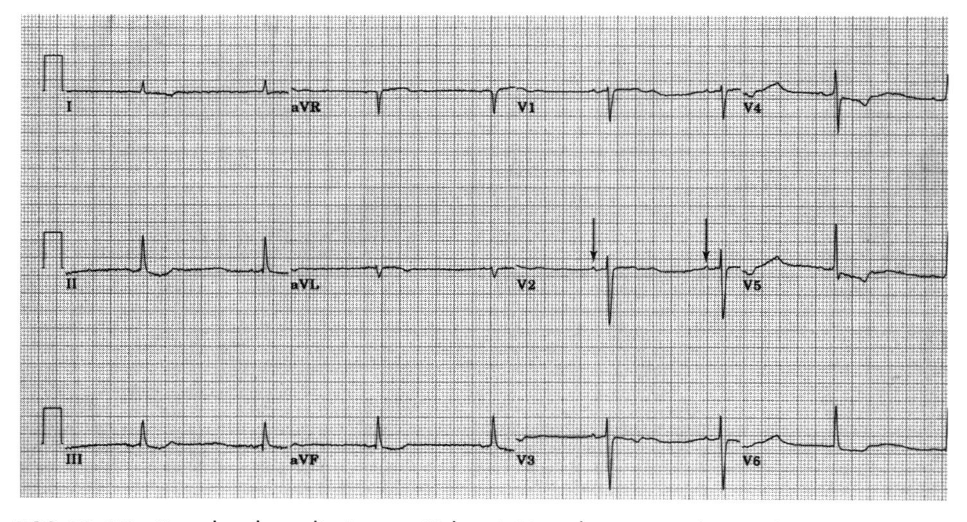

ECG 12–13. Sinus bradycardia (rate < 60 bpm). Note the P waves (*arrows*).

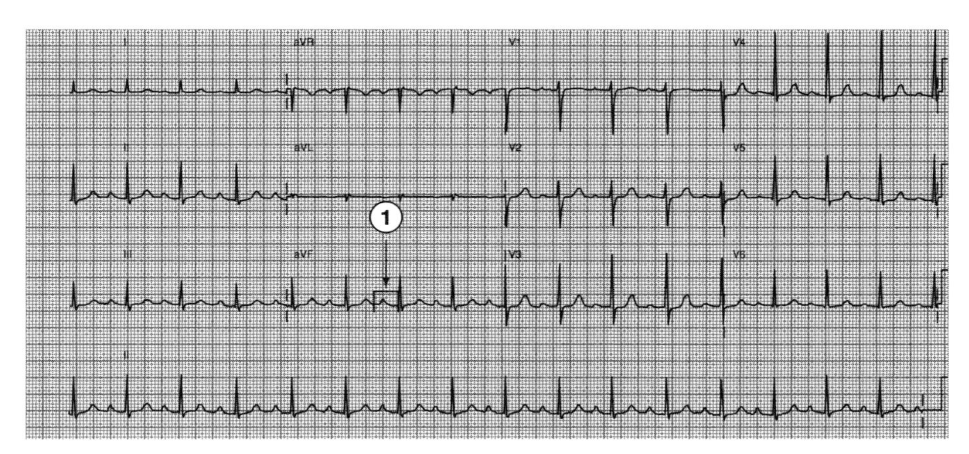

ECG 12–14. First-degree atrioventricular (AV) block. (1) Note the PR interval > 5 small squares.

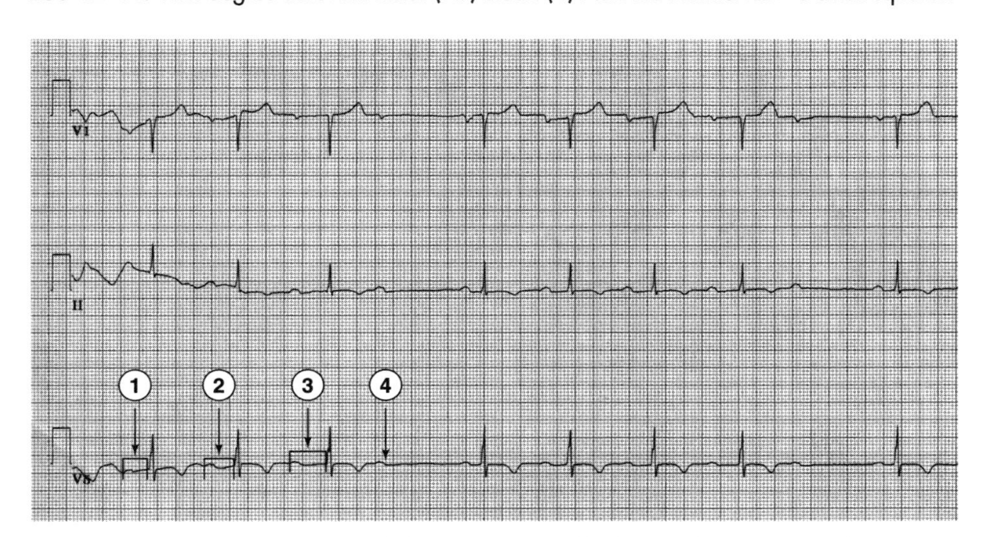

ECG 12–15. (Rhythm strip.) Second-degree type I AV block. Note the progressively increasing PR interval (1, 2, and 3) followed by a dropped QRS (4).

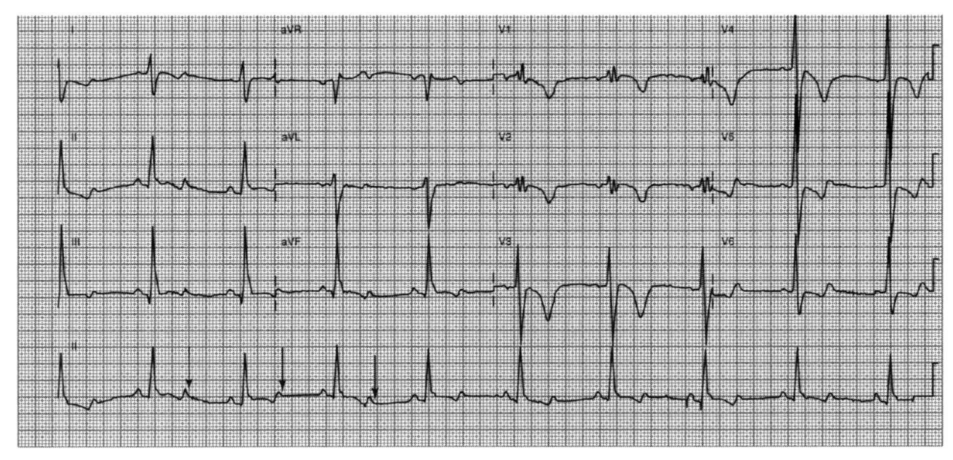

ECG 12–16. Second-degree 2:1 AV block. Note the dropped QRS (*arrows*) after each sinus beat.

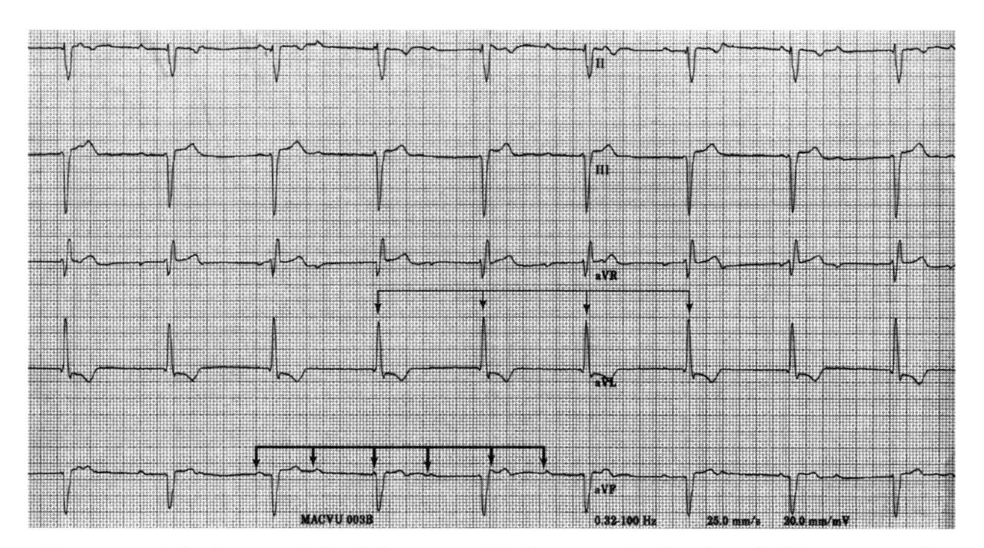

ECG 12–17. (Rhythm strip.) Third-degree AV block. Notice the fixed PP (*bold arrows*) and RR (*arrows*) intervals; however, there is no definite P to R relation.

TRANSIENT ARRHYTHMIAS

You need to have a good grasp of the diagnosis and significance of various transient arrhythmias. You will be frequently informed about patients who reveal arrhythmias on the heart monitors. If the arrhythmia is a few seconds of narrow-complex tachycardia without hemodynamic compromise, you may simply order electrolyte levels and correct them if needed. Ventricular ectopy tends to be of greater concern. If the patient is found to be having very frequent ventricular ectopy or transient (lasting few seconds) runs of ventricular tachycardia, these steps should be followed:

- ❑ Check the patient's electrolyte levels, including magnesium, and correct any abnormality.
- ❑ Determine if the patient has a heart problem and find out if the left ventricular systolic function is compromised. Ventricular ectopy needs to be taken more seriously in patients with left ventricular systolic dysfunction.
- ❑ Determine if the patient has had similar ectopy in the past and see if he or she is taking any antiarrhythmics. For example, it may not be necessary to start the patient on lidocaine if he or she is already receiving amiodarone for similar ectopy.

On the other hand, if you are called about a patient experiencing transient bradycardia without hemodynamic compromise, try to eliminate any iatrogenic causes (mostly drugs) and watch for any more significant episodes. The exceptions are when the patient has high-grade blocks or has ventricular ectopy due to bradycardia. In such situations, you should consider getting an immediate cardiology consult.

COMPUTER READING OF ECGS

Most modern ECG machines provide a simultaneous computerized reading of the ECG. These reports are in no way comparable to the accuracy of a reading by an experienced physician. When at a loss as to how to interpret the ECG, you may consider being guided by this report. However, an experienced person should read the ECG at the earliest chance.

THE MENTOR PROGRAM

A mentor is a faculty member in your training program who has volunteered to guide residents in academic as well as social matters. Most good programs make arrangements for setting residents up with a mentor. The mentors are either assigned to the residents or residents are invited to choose their mentor. Mentorship is a positive tradition in U.S. teaching institutions; however, I have noticed that most IMGs tend to be oblivious of the help that a good mentor can offer. Apart from other things, your mentor can be an authentic resource, providing insights into a new culture.

QUALITIES OF A MENTOR

My discussions with medical students and residents have helped identify several qualities to look for in a mentor:

- Availability. The mentor should be available to you within a reasonable time when you need him or her. There is no point in choosing an academic titan who has no time for mentoring
- Approachability.
- Interest in mentoring. I know several mentors who even give out their home phone numbers to the residents they are mentoring.

- Status. The mentor should preferably have attained a status (academic or financial) that you would like to attain in the years to come.
- On a more selfish note, it is more useful to have a mentor who has good standing in the field that you want to pursue later on. I think this should be a consideration only if the other qualities enumerated above are present.

MEETING YOUR MENTOR

You should call your designated or chosen mentor as soon as possible to set up a time to meet. Most times, a good mentor will be able to initiate a discussion that acquaints both of you with each other. This meeting sets the stage for subsequent, less time-consuming but more useful meetings.

WHAT CAN A GOOD MENTOR DO FOR YOU?

A good mentor is like a good friend. There is no limit or boundary on the matters you can discuss with your mentor. But you should also have respect for the mentor's time and other engagements. Following are some of the areas with which your mentor can help you:

- How to handle problems with other colleagues or staff
- Counseling regarding the future academic plans
- The process of getting a fellowship in the field of your interest
- The stresses of residency as well as the stress of introduction to a new culture

Finally, your mentor can sometimes act as a social springboard.

You should have a clear idea about what you want to get out of a rotation before starting it.

HOW TO GET THE MAXIMUM BENEFIT FROM A ROTATION

The residency program in the United States is divided into 1-month or 4-week time blocks. Each block is called a rotation. You change over to a different department at the end of each rotation. The residency curriculum is designed in such a way to ensure that you receive enough exposure to each department as is mandated by the certifying boards (ABIM in the case of internal medicine). You are likely to rotate through the following departments during your residency:

1. Floor rotation: Here, you take care of the patients admitted in the hospital. These rotations are mandatory.
2. Operating room (OR) rotations, in case of residency in surgical fields.
3. A minimum number of emergency department (ED) rotations are mandatory for residency.
4. Consult rotation: This includes rotations providing consultations for the specialty in which you are doing residency or the consultation service for related subspecialties (e.g., neurology, hematology, and so on, during a medicine residency). You can have a say in choosing different departments for this type of rotations.
5. Critical care rotations, which include the ICU and cardiac care unit (CCU) rotations.
6. Ambulatory care: During this rotation, you mainly see patients in the outpatient (OP) setting. The training acquired during these rotations is likely to be of great help to you later when managing patients in practice. I think typical training is skewed too much in favor of inpatient and critical care training.
7. Electives: As the name implies, these are the rotations that you elect to do. This could be a rotation in a subspecialty of your interest, an extra rotation in the ED, ambulatory care, or critical care rotations. You should choose an elective rotation on the basis of the following considerations:
   a. This is the subject that you are particularly interested in knowing more about.
   b. You think that you need to consolidate your knowledge base for this subject.
   c. You want to pursue a career in this subspecialty or you want to see more before deciding if you want to pursue a career in this specialty.
   d. You want to have the opportunity to work with a particular teacher. That, in turn, could be because you want to have a good recommendation letter from that person.
   e. You want to have hands-on experience with certain procedures that you can learn well in this rotation.

Before you start any rotation, you should spend some time trying to evaluate what you want to gain from this rotation. The Accreditation

Committee for Graduate Medical Education (ACGME) requires that all departments in the programs training residents have a printed curriculum that is given to residents at the start of the rotation. These are mostly nicely written documents that describe what the chief of that department hopes to help you gain from that particular rotation. Sometimes reading this can give you a better idea of what you should expect from a given rotation. You should request a copy of this curriculum at the start of the rotation. The residency is the only time when you can concentrate mainly on the job of learning without thinking about the business aspects of your trade. You should spend this time learning hands on and from others' experience as far as possible. Before starting a rotation, make a list of the goals you want to achieve during that rotation. Examples might include:

- ❑ Learn the procedures that are going to be useful in your practice
- ❑ Learn the topics that are likely to be useful in your line of intended practice
- ❑ Learn to use certain equipment that you are hesitant now to touch
- ❑ Have exposure to a particular patients population

Reevaluate your progress in the middle of the rotation. If you think you are not meeting your goals, talk to your attending or senior resident about your expectations and ask how you can meet them.

CLINICAL EXAMINATION TEST

This is a test that you are required to take during your residency training. It is one of the requirements set by the American Board of Internal Medicine (ABIM). This is somewhat similar to the CSA, the difference being that it takes place during the residency and one of your own teachers conducts the test. For this test, you will be assigned a patient. You are required to perform a history and physical examination in front of the teacher. After this, you discuss the patient with your teacher. The information included throughout this book should help you do well on this clinical exam. Some of the aspects on which you are tested are outlined in Table 12–4.

TABLE 12–4. Areas Evaluated by the Clinical Examination Test

1. History: The ability to elicit all parts of history.
2. Interpersonal skills: This includes the ability to:
   a. Greet patients and introduce yourself at the start of the interview.
   b. Use appropriate eye contact and convey an attitude of interest and respect for the patient.
   c. Extract useful information with open-ended questions.
   d. Recognize emotional content and nonverbal cues from the patient.
3. Physical examination: The examiner is given a proforma with a list of steps to be followed for a thorough examination of each system. He or she will note any steps missed by you. Refer to the discussion earlier in this chapter for more information.
4. Presentation and treatment: This includes the ability to:
   a. Present the patient problem(s) in an organized fashion.
   b. Identify problems and prioritize them.
   c. Understand the pathophysiology and differential diagnosis of major problems.
   d. Select diagnostic tests on the basis of likely yield and risk/benefit issues.
   e. Select an effective treatment plan.

Note: You are graded on the basis of your performance on all four aspects.

EVALUATION

At the end of each rotation, you will be evaluated by your teaching attending. These evaluations become a part of your file. These evaluations are extremely important to the advancement of your career. If you receive good evaluations, you will receive good recommendations—and good recommendations can help your career advancement in the United States. Residents are usually evaluated on the areas listed in Table 12–5.

Just as there are good exam takers, there are also good evaluation takers.

The evaluation form contains headings similar to the items listed in Table 12–5. Residents and interns are evaluated on a scale from 1 to 9 for each quality. There are few blank lines at the end of the form, for your evaluator's comments. The few good or bad comments written here will have more impact than the preceding numerical evaluation. The residency accrediting agency recommends the process of evaluation outlined in Table 12–6.

TABLE 12–5. Areas Evaluated in Each Clinical Rotation

Clinical judgment
Medical knowledge
Clinical skills, including history, physical examination, and procedural skills
Humanistic qualities
Medical care
Attitudes and professional behavior
Overall clinical competence

TABLE 12–6. Recommended Evaluation Procedure for Residents

1. The evaluator should meet the resident during mid-rotation and discuss with the resident his or her progress to that point. The evaluator should indicate the areas in which the resident needs to improve. This should be accompanied by helpful suggestions.
2. At the end of the rotation, the evaluator should sit down with the resident and discuss his or her performance in detail and should give constructive feedback.
3. Both the evaluator and the resident should sign the evaluation form.
4. This evaluation should then be sent to the department chief, who should also read and sign it before putting it in the candidate's file.

HELPFUL INFORMATION

Empower yourself by reading the various publications available from the ABIM.

The ABIM puts out several terrific publications that are available free of charge. You should read them to be sure you understand the meaning of the different terms used in Table 12–5. Following is a list of recommended ABIM publications.

- *Guide to Evaluation of Residents in Internal Medicine*
- *Residents: Evaluating Your Clinical Competence*
- *Attending Physicians: Your Role in Evaluating Residents*
- *Project Professionalism*
- *Guide to Awareness and Evaluation of Humanistic Qualities*

These publications can be requested by calling 800-441-2246 (within the United States) or 215-446-3500, or by e-mail at *request@abim.org*.

Various publications write in detail about the suggested method of appropriate evaluation, but unfortunately, evaluation is not an objective method. There tends to be a lot of room for manipulations. The mental makeup of the evaluator or the outward charms of the resident can heavily influence it. The end of rotation evaluation time can become more of a time for social niceties. You should read the list of things included in the evaluation form as given above and also try to read ABIM publications. On the basis of that knowledge, you should try to cultivate 'eval-taking skills.' It is just like cultivating the examination-taking skills.

In response to my question 'Can you manipulate your evaluation?', the answers were

- Sweet manners can win them all
- Use end of rotation rituals like 'Thanks for being a great teacher' card and end of rotation party
- Presenting mementos can help

The above pointers may help you be more evaluation savvy. But I will strongly recommend that your main thrust should be towards becoming an excellent doctor and learning as much as you can during these years of training.

CHAPTER 13

Some Distinctive Features of the Practice of Medicine in the United States

ETHICS, PATIENT RIGHTS, AND LEGAL ISSUES

Ethics is a dynamic concept. It is potentially influenced by three factors:

1. Patients' expectations and beliefs
2. Physicians' beliefs and cultural background
3. The expectations of the society as a whole

This dynamic quality makes it all the more important for IMGs to know some important facts about the practice of medicine in the United States. In the context of the doctor–patient relationship, ethical decisions should always be made with respect for the patient's beliefs. The physician or the surrogate decision-maker (in the case of a mentally incompetent patient) should avoid projecting his or her own expectations or beliefs onto the patient's situation.

Ethical decisions should be made with respect to patients' beliefs. The physician should avoid projecting his or her own expectations or beliefs onto the patient's situation.

Not infrequently, the ethical and legal considerations of the same problem demand different actions. In such situations, you will have to make morally correct decisions without getting into trouble with the law. Each hospital has an ethics committee and a risk management department. You should ask for their help in making any difficult decisions. An ethics committee may consist of members of the medical profession, members of society, and local religious leaders. The risk management department can advise you about local laws.

As a general rule, a stepwise approach as outlined in Table 13–1 is helpful for most situations involving ethical issues.

TABLE 13–1. A Stepwise Approach to Ethical Decision Making

- ❑ The principles of beneficence (duty to promote good and act in the best interest of the patient and society) and nonmaleficence (duty to do no harm to the patient) should be followed as far as possible.
- ❑ Whenever there is a disagreement between you and the patient or his or her family, make sure that it is not due to their lack of understanding of the situation. Make every effort to answer all of their queries.
- ❑ There may be situations where you are 100 percent sure of the ethical and legal correctness of your stance. Here, you should explain the situation to the patient and family. Never threaten your patient with any legal recourse on your own. If you see something illegal being done, let the legal department handle it.
- ❑ If you still do not succeed in reaching a common ground, you may discuss the situation with your hospital's ethics committee and risk management department.
- ❑ If you are strongly against an action that the patient or his family insists on, you may consider transferring the patient's care to another physician.

ETHICAL ISSUES

Competence

All mentally competent patients should make all decisions about their care decisions. Doctors should not act in a paternalistic manner. In the case of a mentally incompetent patient, you should turn to one of the patient's close family members or significant other. If the patient has designated a legal proxy, that person should make decisions for the patient. Some states specify the order in which family members will serve as surrogates in the absence of patient's directives. If the patient had ever expressed his or her preferences regarding health care decisions to the surrogate, those decisions should be respected. All this may look simpler on paper than in real-life situations. For example, a patient's five adult children may have differing opinions about the care of their father. In such cases, you should always try to assist them in reaching a consensus on the basis of your explanations or group discussion, even if the oldest child (according to the law in some states) can legally make the decision. This is ethically more fair to all the people involved and can also help prevent any of the angry participants from later slapping you with a lawsuit.

Confidentiality

Different states have different laws about the rights of adolescent patients to confidentiality. You should normally encourage the adolescent patient to share the information with his or her parents. Note, however, that if a third party gives information to a doctor about the patient with instructions not to reveal the source of the information to the patient, the physician is not obliged to refrain.

Patient–Physician Relationship

In the absence of a preexisting relationship, you are ethically obliged to take care of a patient only if there is no other physician available or the patient needs emergency care. If your personal beliefs prevent you from providing specific treatment to a patient, you should transfer care to another physician.

Sometimes serious differences arise between a patient and physician, and the physician may want to terminate the professional relationship with the patient. In such cases, you should seriously try to resolve any conflicts before transferring the patient's care to another physician. If you want to transfer care of the patient to another doctor, you should make sure that the patient has alternative arrangement available to him or her. If the patient needs to be physically moved, it is the physician's responsibility to arrange adequate and safe transport.

You should always discuss a patient's condition with him or her, handling the issue of disclosing unpleasant information with great sensitivity.

If you are at risk of contracting an illness while taking care of a patient, you must take the necessary preventive steps. Your workplace is obligated to provide such safety measures to you. It is unethical to refuse care to patients suffering from *any* disease.

You should not stop taking care of a patient just because the patient wants to try an alternative medicine treatment. The patient has the right to choose care. You should ask why the patient is seeking alternative care, to determine if it is due to the patient's dissatisfaction with the present care.

You should avoid taking care of close friends, family members, and employees. Also avoid the temptation to give "curbside" advice to friends.

Impaired Physician

If a physician feels that he or she has an impairment that may interfere with the ability to provide proper care to his or her patients, the physician should stop being the care provider. The physician should also seek help from a qualified source. If you suspect a colleague of being impaired, you have the ethical duty to report the person to the higher authorities. This may be easier said than done.

End of Life Issues

Patients suffering from terminal illnesses have the right to autonomy and self-determination. Their symptoms should be adequately controlled, with good pain control being one of the examples. A physician need not provide treatment he or she feels is likely to be totally futile. But here again, the matter should be resolved through discussion with the patient and family. If the discussion fails and you feel strongly against the line of management, you may consider transferring care.

Advanced Directives

An advanced directive allows the patient to indicate his or her preference for care in the event he or she becomes incompetent at some point in time. This is an example of the patient's right to self-determination. A patient can also legally designate another person as a surrogate decision-maker or give that person power of attorney. This person is then authorized to make decisions on behalf of the patient in case the patient is unable to do so.

Advanced directives should be as detailed as possible. As an example, the physician should counsel the patient to specify whether he or she would want to be given IV fluids or artificial feeding as a life-prolonging measure in the event of a terminal illness.

A "Do not resuscitate" order (DNR order) is a wish expressed by the patient to refrain from providing cardiopulmonary resuscitation to him or her in the event of cardiorespiratory arrest. The physician should encourage patients with serious illnesses and those in advanced old age to indicate their wishes concerning resuscitation. DNR orders become a part of the patient's records after discussion between the physician and the patient or his or her surrogate. Short of cardiorespiratory arrest, the patient with DNR order should be treated exactly like anyone else. In some situations, the health care team may feel that carrying out resuscitation measures for a particular patient will be futile, but the patient has no DNR orders on file. In such cases, the team may respond with slow or half-hearted efforts. This is called a "slow code" (Gazelle, G., N Engl Med 1998; 338:467–469). While it is a rare occurrence, it is also unethical.

The preceding information on ethical issues is intended to provide examples of situations you are likely to face in medical practice. Individual situations will require their own decisions and actions. When in doubt as to the proper course of action, seek guidance from the appropriate hospital staff.

LEGAL ISSUES

Legal issues are an important concern for physicians practicing in the U.S. All active decisions should be made after discussions with your team. A few useful tips are provided in Table 13–2.

DOCUMENTATION

Proper documentation is the responsibility of every patient care provider, and it has legal implications for providers in the event of a lawsuit by the patient. Several tips for ensuring adequate documentation are provided in Table 13–3.

TABLE 13–2. Tips for Providing Legally Defensible Care

- ❑ Always act in the best interest of the patient. Be the patient's advocate.
- ❑ Keep the communication lines open between you and the patient as well as the patient's family.
- ❑ In the event that a mistake is made in the care of a patient, communicate it to the patient or the patient's relatives. Do not try to cover up mistakes.
- ❑ Always give discussion your best shot in cases where you and the patient or family are at odds over the course of treatment.
- ❑ Always listen to the patient or family's complaints or concerns even if they seem to be irrelevant or frivolous.
- ❑ Always provide proper documentation in the chart. Any discussion or treatment decision should be written in the chart. As a resident, whenever you see another team's patient on call day, write a note indicating why you were called to see the patient and what actions you took.

TABLE 13–3. Tips for Ensuring Proper Documentation

- ❑ Always date and time your notes.
- ❑ Never try to fit your afterthoughts in between lines previously written by you. This can be seen as an effort to alter the record. Additional comments should be written under the heading "addendum."
- ❑ Never write negative statements about other members of the health care team in the chart. This can prove harmful to you as well as the other person.
- ❑ If you want to remove a statement you wrote from the chart, run a single line through it. Do not try to black it out to prevent anyone else from deciphering what you wrote.
- ❑ Never scratch out anything written by someone else. Sometimes the team as a whole may decide that the line of action should be different from what another person wrote. In this case, simply write a new statement explaining the new action.

SEXUAL HARASSMENT

Sometimes seemingly benign actions at the workplace can constitute legal grounds for a case of sexual harassment. Residency training programs should educate their trainees about the concept of sexual harassment in the workplace. If you do not receive information on this topic as a part of your regular training, you should request it from your program director.

EVIDENCE-BASED MEDICINE

Recently a great deal of attention has been given to the issue of evidence-based medicine. The importance of this focus is underscored by the decision to include items testing examinees' understanding of simple statistics on the board exams. You will need to understand several frequently used terms and be able to critically evaluate the medical literature.

DIAGNOSTIC PERFORMANCE

Sensitivity and specificity are two characteristics of a test. Each is expressed as a percentage. This percentage is the same regardless of the pretest probability of a disease in an individual or the prevalence of a disease in any population. But the absolute number of patients with a false positive or negative test is affected by the prevalence of the disease.

Sensitivity

The sensitivity of a test is the number of persons who actually have a disease out of the total number of persons who are classified as having the disease on the basis of a positive (abnormal) test. As previously noted, this is expressed as percentage. As an example, let us say 200 patients are tested and 100 patients out of this 200-patient sample have the disease that the test is designed to detect. If the test is positive in 95 out of 100 patients with the disease, the sensitivity of the test is 95 percent. The sensitivity of a test can be calculated with the help of the 2×2 table shown in Figure 13–1.

$$\text{Sensitivity} = \frac{\text{Total number of persons with the disease who have positive test}}{\text{Total number of individuals with the disease}} = \frac{a}{a + c}$$

Test	Persons with disease	Persons without disease	
Positive	a	b	a + b
Negative	c	d	c + d
	a + c = no. of persons with dz.	b + d = no. of persons without the disease (dz.)	

FIGURE 13–1.

Better sensitivity is a desirable characteristic of a test when it is used for screening for a disease. A test with a high sensitivity can be used to rule out a disease because it is likely to be abnormal in most of the patients with the disease.

Let us go back to the earlier example of 200 patients. We have completely ignored the other half of the group (those without the disease) while calculating sensitivity. Although the test we have examined has good sensitivity, it may also be abnormal in 50 percent of the patients without the disease (false positive). In such a situation, while the test is successfully detecting patients with the disease, it also is giving wrong information leading to unnecessary additional studies or, worse still, unnecessary treatment in 50 percent of the patients without the disease. This characteristic of the test is addressed in specificity.

Specificity

Specificity is a measure of the percentage of the persons without the disease who have a normal test. In the example above, if the test is negative in 92 of the 100 patients without the disease, the test has a specificity of 92 percent.

$$\text{Specificity} = \frac{\text{Number of persons with no disease and a negative test}}{\text{Total number of disease-free individuals}}$$

$$= d/b + d \text{ (See Fig. 13–1)}$$

A test with high specificity is desirable when you want to be reasonably sure that a person with an abnormal test result *has* the disease. A test with high specificity is useful for “ruling in” a disease.

Sensitivity and specificity are general statements about a test; they do not give help that is tailored for individual situations.

Positive and Negative Predictive Value

These values tell us about the chances of a person having or not having the disease when the test is positive or negative, respectively. Using the 2×2 table in Figure 13–1, the predictive value is as follows:

Positive predictive value (Predictive value of a Positive test)

$$= \frac{\text{Number of persons with the disease and a positive test}}{\text{Total number of persons with a positive test}}$$
$$= a/a + b$$

Negative predictive value (Predictive value of a negative test)

$$= \frac{\text{Number of persons without the disease and with a negative test}}{\text{Total number of persons with a negative test}}$$
$$= d/c + d$$

The two values above interact with the pretest probability to give us the positive and negative predictive values in individual situations.

The pretest probability of a disease refers to the chance of the patient having a disease prior to the performance of a particular test. This is decided by a doctor on the basis of the history, physical examination of the patient, any previous test results, and knowledge of various aspects of the disease. The pretest probability of the same patient having ischemic colitis may be put at 1 percent by an experienced surgeon and 90 percent by a physician not well versed in this disease. The pretest probability of 90 percent in this example means that, according to the second physician, if there were 1,000 *exactly similar* patients with similar presentations, 900 out of them would prove to have ischemic colitis.

A physician has to start with the pretest probability in order to be guided by further tests, despite this being a changeable number. Thus, we can use the numbers in a 2×2 table to calculate the predictive value of a test. Let us suppose that we schedule a test for the diagnosis of ischemic colitis in the patient described above. Let us further suppose this test has a sensitivity and a specificity of 80 percent and 90 percent, respectively. Using a total of 1,000 patients and a 90 percent probability, we will construct the 2×2 table shown in Figure 13–2.

90% Pretest Probability

	Persons with disease	Persons without disease	
Positive test	720	10	730
Negative test	180	90	270
	900	100	

FIGURE 13–2.

$$\text{Positive predictive value} = a/a + b = 720/730 = 98.6\%$$
$$\text{Negative predictive value} = d/c + d = 90/270 = 33.3\%$$

Now, if we design a 2 × 2 table using a 1 percent probability, the calculation will be:

$$\text{Positive predictive value} = a/a{+}b = 8/107 = 7.5\%$$
$$\text{Negative predictive value} = d/c{+}d = 891/893 = 99.8\%$$

The predictive value of this same test is different in the same patient with different pretest probability given by two examiners despite the sensitivity and specificity of the test remaining the same.

Likelihood Ratio (LR)

Ideally one desires to have a test with both high sensitivity and high specificity. In real-life situations, however, one frequently has to choose from several available tests with no clear winner in terms of both sensitivity and specificity. One criterion for choosing a test is by calculating the LR, which depends on the sensitivity and specificity of the test. The LR of a positive test is the ratio of the probability of a positive test when the disease is present to the probability of a positive test when the disease is not present. This can be stated as:

$$\text{LR of a positive test} = \frac{\text{Sensitivity}}{100\% - \text{specificity}}.$$

Similarly, the LR of a negative test is the ratio of the probability of a negative test when the disease is present to the probability of a negative test when disease is not present. This can be stated as:

$$\text{LR of a negative test} = \frac{100\% - \text{sensitivity}}{\text{Specificity}}.$$

Pretest Probability

This is the proportion of patients who have the disease before the test is carried out. According to Figure 13–1, it is $a+c/a+b+c+d$.

Pretest Odds

This is defined as the ratio of probability of a disease to 1 − probability of disease. It can be stated as:

$$\frac{\text{Pretest probability}}{1-\text{pretest probability}}.$$

Posttest Odds

This is the odds of patient having a disorder after the test, or Pretest odds × LR.

Posttest Probability

This is the proportion of persons with a *given* test result who have the disorder in question. In other words, it tells you the probability of a person having a disease on the basis of the test result. It can be stated as:

$$\frac{\text{Posttest odds}}{1+\text{postest odds}}.$$

A nomogram published in the *New England Journal of Medicine* (Fagan TJ: Nomogram for Bayes's Theorem, N Engl J Med 1975;293:257) can help you obtain posttest probability from the known pretest probability and LR without making lengthy calculations.

Odds Ratio

This is a summary statistic that gives a measure of association between an etiological factor and a condition. The odds ratio gives the odds of having a risk factor if the condition is present as compared to having a risk factor if the condition is not present. Using the example of smoking and lung cancer, we can make another 2×2 table (Fig. 13–3).

The odds of being a smoker for a patient who has lung cancer are:

$$\frac{\text{Patients with lung cancer who smoke}}{\text{Patients with lung cancer who do not smoke}} = a/c.$$

The odds of being a smoker for a patient who does not have lung cancer, according to Figure 13–3 are b/d. Thus,

$$\text{Odds ratio} = \frac{a/c}{b/d}.$$

Relative Risk

This is the ratio between the probability of *developing a condition if the risk is present* and the probability of developing the same condition if the risk factor is not present. As compared to relative risk, the odds ratio is the ratio between the probability of *having a risk factor if the condition is present* and the probability of having a risk factor if the condition is not present.

Referring again to Figure 13–3, the risk of developing lung cancer in smokers is $a/a+b$. The risk of developing cancer in nonsmokers is $c/c+d$. Thus,

$$\text{Relative risk} = \frac{a/a+b}{c/c+d}.$$

A relative risk of 15 will imply that the smokers are 15 times more likely to have lung cancer as compared to nonsmokers.

	Lung cancer	No lung cancer
Smoking	a	b
Not smoking	c	d
	a + c	b + d

FIGURE 13–3.

Relative Risk Reduction (RRR)

The RRR can be stated as follows:

$$\frac{\text{Event rate in the experimental group - event rate in the control group}}{\text{Event rate in the control group}}$$

Absolute Risk Reduction (ARR)

The ARR is defined simply as the event rate in the experimental group minus the event rate in the control group.

Number Needed to Treat (NNT)

This is the number of patients who need to be treated before one intended favorable result be achieved. It is derived from the formula 1/ARR. The NNT should be rounded off to nearest whole number. This number may serve as a guide as to whether an intervention is cost-effective or even worth the effort, because each action has some expense as well as side effects attached to it.

DIFFERENT PHASES OF TRIAL

All therapies proposed for use in U.S. medical practice must undergo rigorous clinical trials, which consist of three phases. Phase I is the initial phase of administering the therapy in question to human subjects. This is used to establish a dosage regimen and also to watch for any potential toxicities. Phase II includes small controlled or uncontrolled trials carried out as a preface to randomized control trials. Phase III trials are undertaken after the data from the initial studies has been studied.

DIFFERENT TYPES OF STUDIES AND TRIALS

Case Control Study

This is a retrospective study, as illustrated by the following example. You are a researcher who hypothesizes that diabetics may be at higher risk of developing coronary artery disease (CAD). You look at the clinic charts of 3,000 diabetic patients seen in your hospital to see how many of them have CAD. Then you compare this rate to that in the nondiabetic population.

This type of study has at least two advantages: (1) It is easier to do and less time-consuming than other types of studies; and (2) it is useful for studying rare diseases. The main objection to such studies is that they are prone to biases and methodological errors.

This type of study should not always be brushed aside as inferior, however. There may be some types of phenomena that can only be studied with this design. Sometimes a case control study may be the initial step toward more immaculate studies to prove an extremely important observation.

Cohort Study

This is a prospective study. These studies provide a better understanding of the effect of an etiological factor on multiple outcomes. There are two types of cohort studies:

1. In the first type, the patients with a given factor are followed to observe the outcome. Returning to the earlier example, for cohort study the patients with diabetes would be followed for the appearance of the CAD. You may have to follow these patients for years before you can decide whether there is an association between diabetes and CAD. These studies are expensive and time consuming.
2. The second type is called a nonconcurrent cohort study. Suppose you want to study the association of high cholesterol with CAD. A group of patients have cholesterol readings from 20 years ago. These data can be used in a cohort study as long as the identification of individuals for study and control groups is done without knowledge of whether the condition under study has developed.

Both case control and cohort studies are observational studies.

Randomized Clinical Trial

This is a highly respected design. Here, individuals are randomly assigned to a study or control group. The population included in the study (study or control group) is evaluated prior to the study for inclusion and exclusion criteria.

Meta-analysis

This is a method for combining information from different investigations. This type of analysis is very attractive as it tries to give us a gist of different studies on a subject. The shortcomings are that a given analysis may not include all the relevant studies or may include too many poorly designed studies.

STATISTICAL SIGNIFICANCE

The investigations are usually performed on a subset of larger population known as a sample. There is always the question of whether similar results would be obtained if the whole of a population were studied or if a different subset of the population were selected. Another question is whether the chance selection could have generated some unusual findings in the study sample. For this, statistical significance testing is done. Following are some important concepts in this field.

Null Hypothesis

This is the assumption that no true difference exists between the control and study groups. The null hypothesis in an earlier example on page 260 will be that there is no difference in the prevalence of CAD between diabetics and non-diabetics.

Alternative Hypothesis

This is the hypothesis that disagrees with the null hypothesis. If the null hypothesis is rejected as a result of the evidence in a study, the alternative hypothesis is the conclusion. In a simplistic way, it states the objective of the study. Returning once again to the example on page 260, alternative hypothesis may state "diabetics are known to have increased vascular complications so we hypothesize that they may have greater chances of getting CAD as compared to non-diabetics."

Type I Error

This is the error that occurs when a null hypothesis is falsely rejected. In simple terms, a difference is found between the study and control groups when none exists.

Type II Error

This is the error that occurs when no difference is found between the study and control groups although one actually does exist.

P Value

This is the measure of the statistical significance of an observation. Traditionally, a *P* value of less than .05 is thought to be significant. The word "significant" here means that the collected data has sufficient evidence against the null hypothesis. A *P* value of less than 0.05 means that an observation is accepted as significant if there is less than a 5 percent chance of a finding occurring purely by chance. This is an arbitrarily set number. If the *P* value for a study is less than .07, the chance of an unusual finding happening purely by chance is less than 7 in 100, or 7 percent. If the *P* value is less than .008, the chances of an unusual finding happening purely by chance is less than 8 in 1,000 or 0.8 percent. The *P* value concept is not free of fallacies, and the value of less than .05 should not be taken as gospel. (For those who are interested, a good article is: Goodman, S.N., Towards evidence based medical statistics. 1: p value fallacy. Ann Intern Med 1999;130:995–1004.)

HELPFUL HINTS

A few important points in the context of evidence-based medicine follow.

You must critically evaluate all research data before applying it to your practice of medicine.

- It is important that doctors know the latest advances in medicine, but it is of paramount importance that they accumulate a basic databank about common diseases.
- Different people can interpret the same statistical data in different ways. Never let anyone lead you by the finger on the basis of a "great, well-designed study done by an expert." You should evaluate the soul of the study and try to imagine how it will translate into care of your patients.
- Always determine whether the study population is representative of your patient population.
- Give due respect to the experience of your professors while continuing to incorporate new advancements into your practice style.
- Never let yourself be psyched out by colleagues who blurt out information about many studies (down to their authors) to support their point. First, they may be using any names that come to mind just to impress and overwhelm you. Second, in their enthusiasm to make

their point, they may give more importance to poorly designed studies while ignoring better studies that oppose their point of view.

- Some reputable agencies publish clinical practice guidelines for specific diseases. These are useful resources. For instance, ACP-ASIM publishes guidelines that can be requested by calling 800-523-1546 (in the United States), ext. 2600. They also have a Web site at *www.acponline.org*. AHCPR guidelines can be found on the Web at *www.ahcpr.org*. Some subspecialty organizations also publish guidelines from time to time.
- Read journals such as the *ACP Journal Club* that talk about recent papers, with analysis by an expert.
- Try to read a good book on statistics. I found the following book to be an enjoyable read: Riegelman R, Hirsch R: *Studying a study and testing a test*, 3rd ed. Boston: Little, Brown, 1996.
- *The Journal of American Medical Association* (*JAMA*) publishes a series of articles that I have found to be very useful in analyzing the available literature. It is a continuing series published under title "Users' Guides to the Medical Literature." You should be able to locate the entire series by searching for this title (without the quotes) in MEDLINE with *JAMA* as the chosen journal (see the next section for the tips on how to use MEDLINE). Some of the articles included in this series are:
    a. Barrett A, et al: Users' guides to the medical literature: XVI. How to use guidelines and recommendations about screening. Evidence-based medicine working group. JAMA 1999 Jun 2;281(21) 2029–2035.
    b. Dans AL, et al: Users' guides to the medical literature: XIV. How to decide on the applicability of clinical trial results to your patient. Evidence-based medicine working group. JAMA 1998 Feb 18;279(7):545–549.
    c. Oxman, AD, et al: Users' guides to the medical literature. I. How to get started. The evidence-based medicine working group. JAMA 1993 Nov 3;270(17):2093–2095.

COMPUTERS IN MEDICINE

To most of us, the word "computer" has become synonymous with personal computer. According to the standard dictionary definition, however, a computer is "a programmable electronic device that can store, retrieve, and process data." Using this latter definition, I think everyone in this day and age has used some type of gadget that relies on computer principles. Computers continue to have a great impact on every aspect of the practice of medicine in the United States. Following are several suggestions that are important for IMGs:

- Do not get psyched out just because someone mentions the word "computer" to you. The slogan and goal of the continuing development of computer technology is "user friendliness." If computers were too difficult for the average person to master, they would never have become integrated into the simple activities of daily living of most of the human race. Every workplace should orient its new employees to its computer system. It should take you only a short time to learn this system.
- The ability to type fast is a definite advantage in using the computer. Learn how to type.
- At the start of your residency, your ability to carry out a literature search on the computer can help you impress people. Many of us, however, have never used MEDLINE before coming to the United States.
- PowerPoint® is one of the software programs that can help you develop great slide presentations. You can learn this once you begin your residency. Most hospital libraries should have it.
- More and more hospitals are computerizing their patient records, which has raised the issue of possible breaches of patient confidentiality. This is a dynamic field at the time of writing of this book. You should keep this issue in mind and see how your workplace deals with it.

The last part of this chapter will deal with the following areas: how to perform a MEDLINE search, how to get started on the Internet, and strategies for working with highly informed patients.

MEDLINE® SEARCH

MEDLINE is the National Library of Medicine's bibliographical database on the Internet. It is used for doing literature searches. This database covers the fields of medicine, nursing, dentistry, veterinary medicine, the health care system, and the preclinical sciences. This is a very important tool for doing research on any subject in health care. The main advantages of this search tool are that the information is updated frequently, and it can be accessed any time of the day or night through a computer. As an example, if you want to find the latest and best treatment for HIV, it is best to seek the latest information published in a high-quality journal. MEDLINE provides an easy way to browse for available information on a topic of interest.

It is very important to learn how to do MEDLINE search efficiently.

At the time of writing of this book, MEDLINE:

- Contains citations and abstracts from over 3,900 journals

- Contains over 9 million records dating back to 1966
- Adds approximately 33,000 new citations each month
- However, keep in mind that is does *not* include every single article published in the world.

MEDLINE's web address is *www.nlm.nih.gov/databases/freemedl.html*. Similar to other Web pages on the Internet, the site is set up with several button-like areas, called tabs. Clicking on the different tabs enables you to perform different functions.

MEDLINE is accessed through two search engines called Internet Grateful Med (IGM) and PubMed. The user can choose to use either of them by clicking on either tab. I will explain both of them. As with any other practical manual, the information in the following pages can be better used while actually working on the computer.

Internet Grateful Med

Once you get to this site, you should click on the "search MEDLINE" tab. The left-hand portion of the screen will list the different databases available. MEDLINE is the first on the list, and that is what you will use most of the time. But it is important to be aware of others on the list. Some of them are:

- AIDSLINE
- AIDSDRUGS
- BIOETHICSLINE
- TOXLINE

Once you click on the MEDLINE tab, the screen shown in Figure 13–4 will appear.

Refer to Figure 13–4 as you read the following descriptions of this screen, starting from the top.

- The "*i*" icon can take you to the help menu.
- "Perform Search" tab will perform a search according to the parameters you set.
- "Find MeSH" finds the word for the search term that you type in the box. MESH® stands for medical subject headings. MeSH is the National Library of Medicine's controlled vocabulary thesaurus. It is used to index the articles in the MEDLINE database. Whenever you enter a search term in the box, you should search for its MeSH term by clicking on this tab. You can choose the term that is identical to your

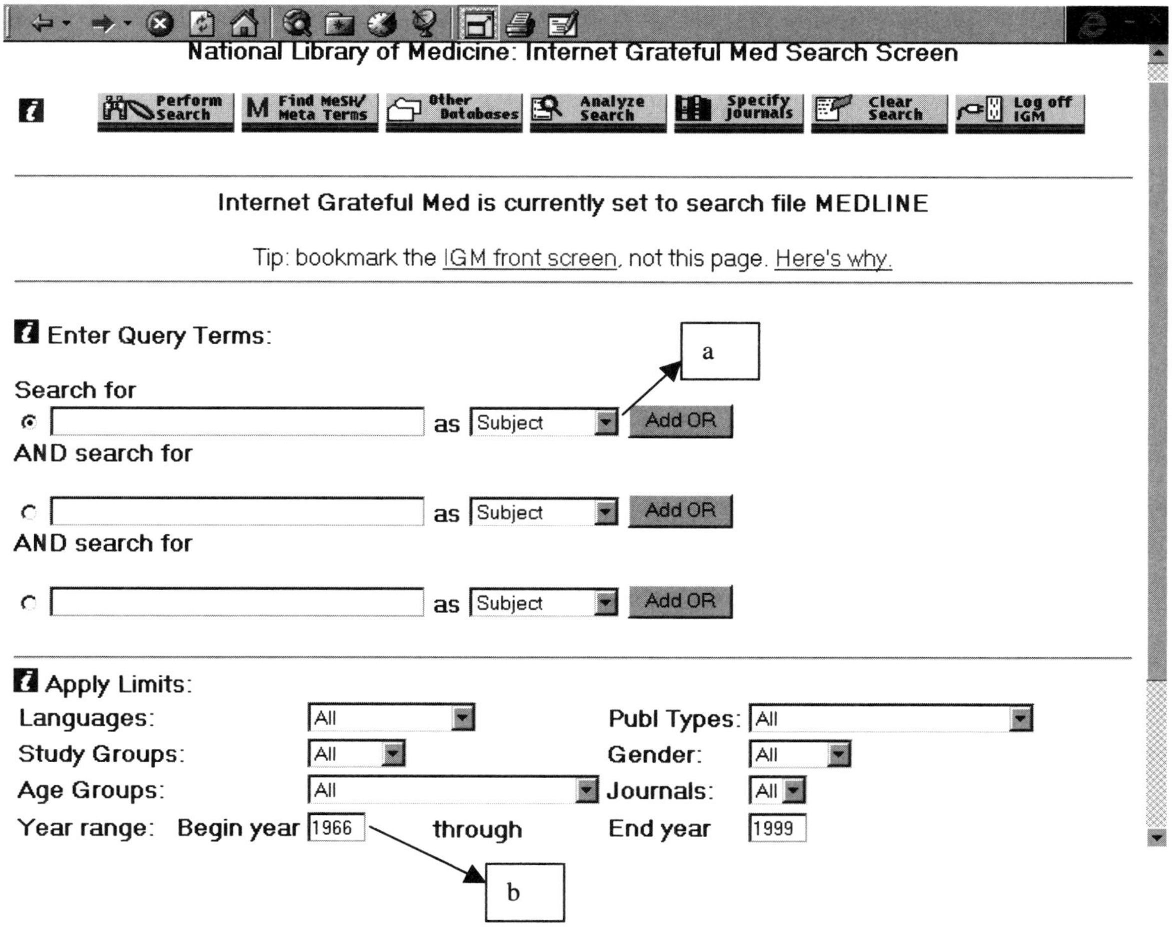

FIGURE 13–4.

term by checking the box to its left. After this, you should click on "Continue Formulating Search." This will give you a choice to "Select Qualifier," which means you can choose whether you want the articles focused on etiology, therapy, or another option from the choice of qualifiers. Then you can return to the search screen.

- "Other Databases" takes you to other databases (apart from MEDLINE) such as AIDSLINE.
- "Specify Journals" helps you search for articles in only the journals you have chosen. After you click on this tab, you will see the screen shown in Figure 13–5. You should type the name of the journal in the empty box. Then you can click on the "Find Alphabetic" or "Find Keyword" tabs. This will give

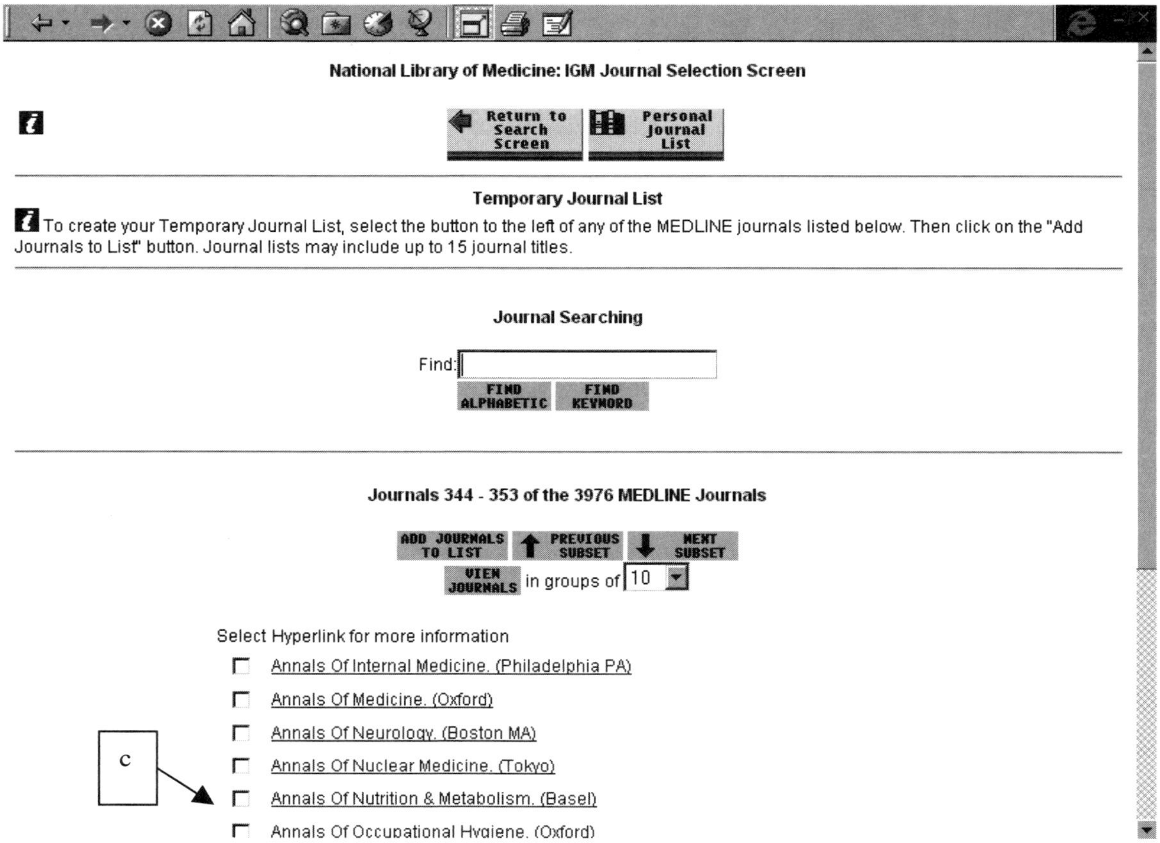

National Library of Medicine: IGM Journal Selection Screen

Return to Search Screen | Personal Journal List

Temporary Journal List

To create your Temporary Journal List, select the button to the left of any of the MEDLINE journals listed below. Then click on the "Add Journals to List" button. Journal lists may include up to 15 journal titles.

Journal Searching

Find:

FIND ALPHABETIC | FIND KEYWORD

Journals 344 - 353 of the 3976 MEDLINE Journals

ADD JOURNALS TO LIST | PREVIOUS SUBSET | NEXT SUBSET

VIEW JOURNALS in groups of 10

Select Hyperlink for more information

- Annals Of Internal Medicine. (Philadelphia PA)
- Annals Of Medicine. (Oxford)
- Annals Of Neurology. (Boston MA)
- Annals Of Nuclear Medicine. (Tokyo)
- Annals Of Nutrition & Metabolism. (Basel)
- Annals Of Occupational Hygiene. (Oxford)

c

FIGURE 13–5.

you a list of journals (c). You should check the box adjacent to the desired journal. You can add multiple journals to the list by repeating the same steps. After this, you should click on the "Return to Search Screen" tab to continue with the search process.

- "Clear Search" clears the parameters specified. After this you can enter new parameters, including new search terms.
- "Log off IGM" lets you disconnect from Internet Grateful Med.
- Continuing with the screen shown in Figure 13–4, you will find three boxes for entering the search terms. These boxes are preceded by the phrase "Search for" to allow you to add more than one search term. For example, if you want to see the articles written about penicillamine use in rheumatoid

arthritis, you can add rheumatoid arthritis in one box and penicillamine in a second box. You can also add both terms in the same box using Boolean logic, as explained later.

- There is a smaller box on the right. In Figure 13–4, it has the word "subject" in it. If you click on the scroll down button (a), you can search by subject, author, or title. To search by author, you should either write the last name followed, after a space, by the initials, or the initials followed by last name in the search box. The search by title is useful when you want to look for a specific article whose title is known to you.
- In the "Apply Limits" block, several qualifiers can be specified from the scroll-down menus in different boxes. If you choose not to apply limits, "All" is the default value, and the default year range is 1966 to the current year.

  a. You can choose to search only for the articles written in a particular language. Note, however, that even articles written in other languages are listed in English in the database.

  b. Under "Publ Types," you can specify if, for example, you only want to look for the review articles or randomized control trials on the search subject.

  c. "Study Groups" lets you choose whether you want articles about research involving humans or animals.

  d. You can also choose studies involving different age groups or gender.

  e. Unless you specify the journals, as explained earlier, all journals will be searched.

  f. You can change the year range in the boxes (b) shown in Figure 13–4. This is useful when, say, you want to search for papers published within the last 10 years.

After you give command to perform the search, the browser will search for all the articles fitting the characteristics you have specified. The results are displayed as shown in Figure 13–6. For each result, the tab on the left, "Full Citation," will take you to the full description (not the original article) of the particular article. You can look at detailed reports on each result individually or you can select the results of interest by clicking on square boxes on the left. In this way, you can look at all of the selected results all at once. "Related articles" will allow

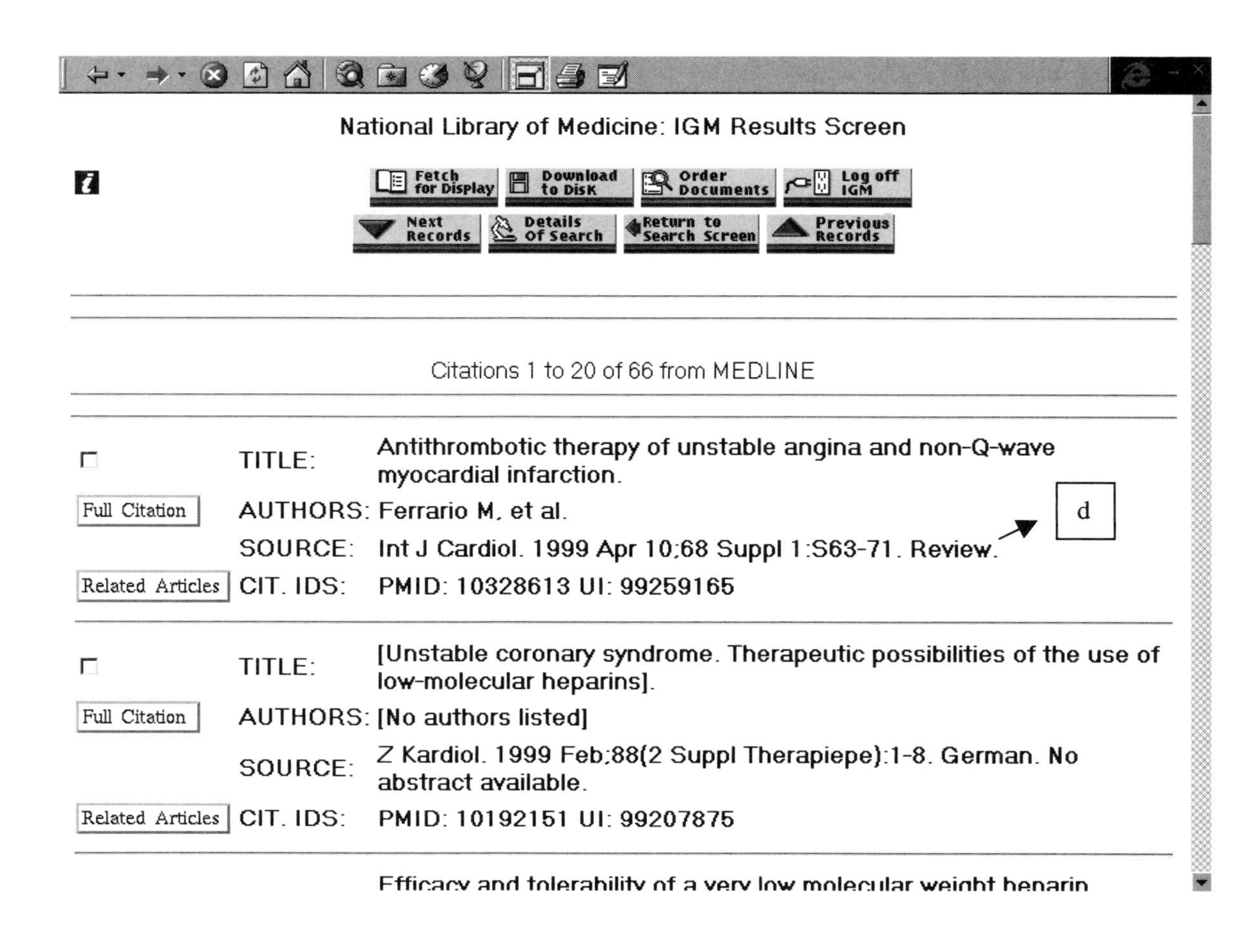

FIGURE 13–6.

you to browse for similar articles. The area labeled (d) will read "No abstract available" if there is none there.

The functions of the tabs on the top of the screen in Figure 13–6 are as follows:

- "Fetch for Display" displays the full citation of all or selected (if selections are made) results on the page.
- "Download to Disk" helps you download and save the results of your search onto your floppy disk.
- "Order Documents" lets you order documents in return for payment. You have to have an account for this. You should talk to your librarian for any article requirements.
- "Log off IGM," "Next Records," "Previous Records," and "Return to search Screen" are self-explanatory
- "Details of Search" gives you the details of the search process done by the browser. I did a search for unstable angina and

low molecular weight heparin, the details of which are shown in Figure 13–7.

The preceding information should help you to carry out an effective literature search. You should choose your own topics for a practice search to help familiarize yourself with the search process.

PubMed

This is another browser for searching MEDLINE. Once you have clicked on "PubMed" on the MEDLINE page, you will go to the PubMed main page, as shown in Figure 13–8. Refer to the column on the left-hand side of the screen in Figure 13–8 as you read the following descriptions of some of the important tabs.

- By clicking on "Advanced Search," you can perform a more specific search (see later discussion).
- "Clinical Queries" is a useful tool when you want to find selected topics on a question. Once you click on this item, the screen shown in Figure 13–9 will appear. You then have

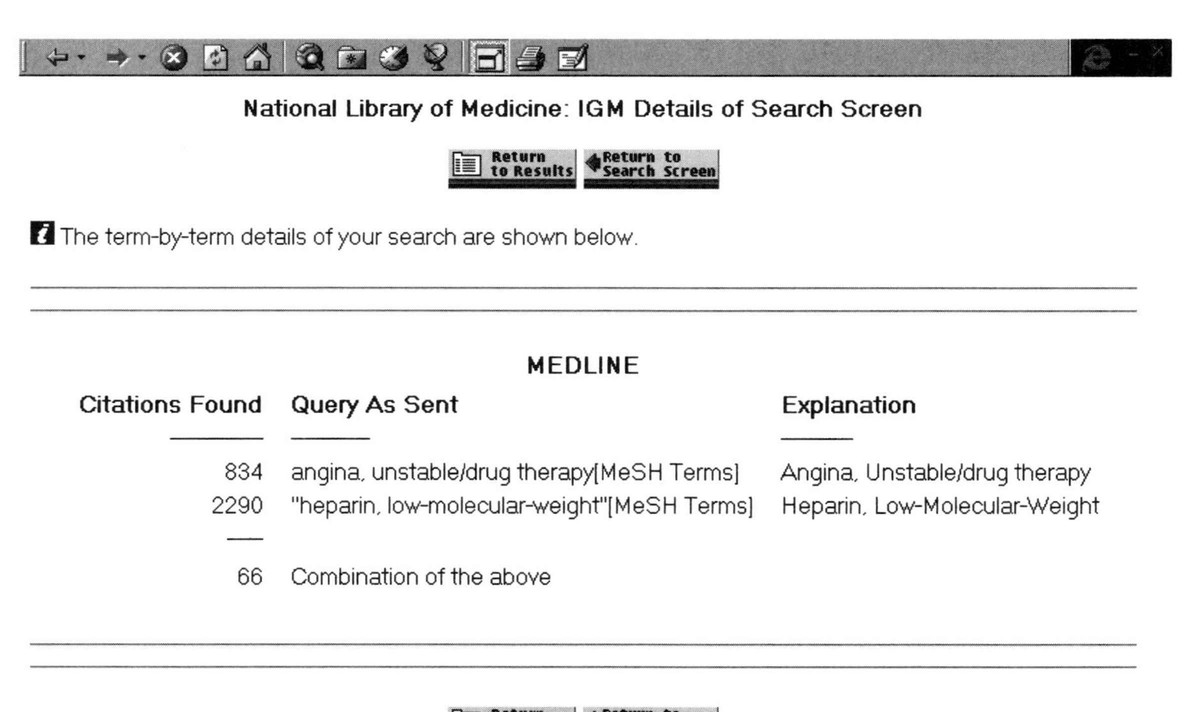

FIGURE 13–7.

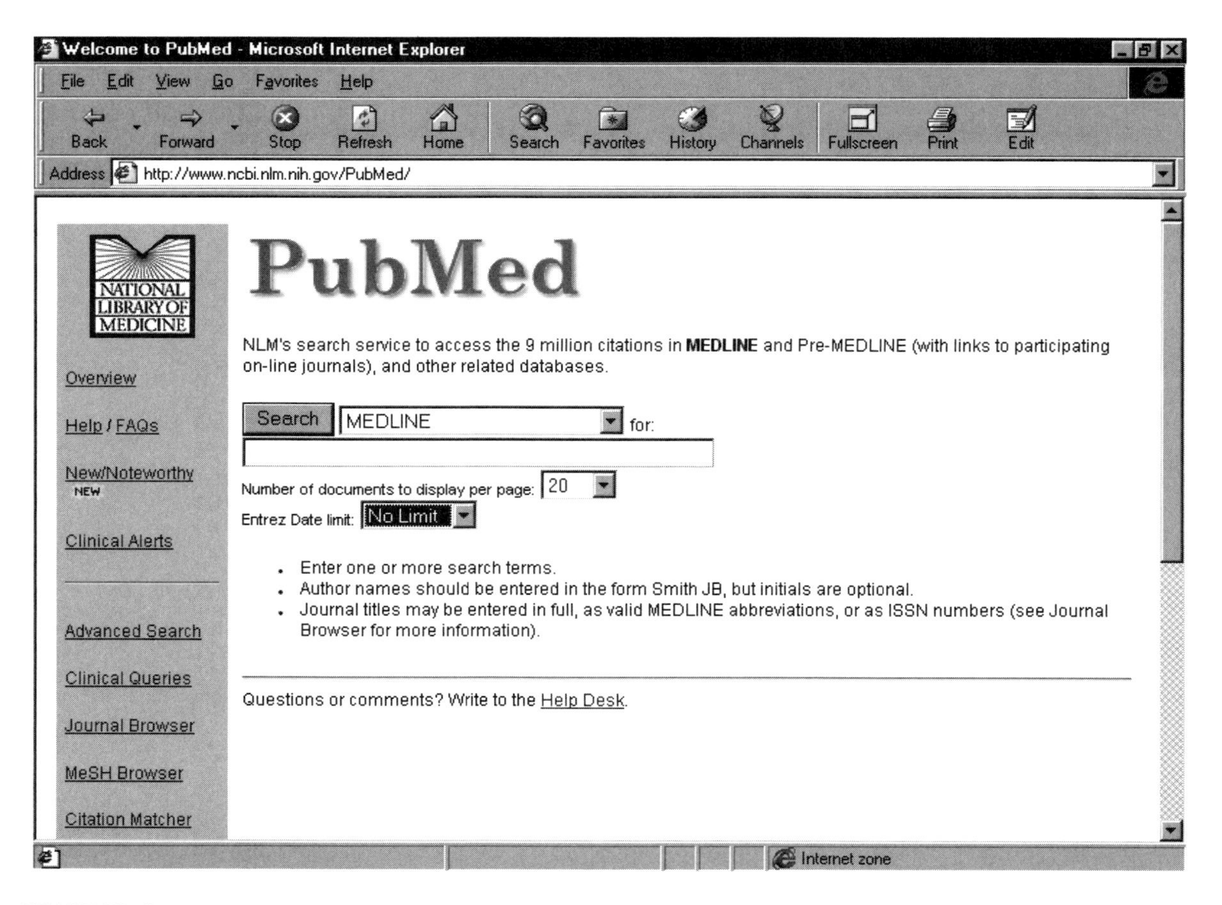

FIGURE 13–8.

to make a selection in the columns "Category" and "Emphasis." As an example, I wondered whether there were any papers addressing the prognostic value of dobutamine stress echo. The result gave me 39 selected articles.

- "Journal Browser" lets you select a particular journal. It also has links to the Web sites of some journals.
- "MeSH Browser" lets you find the MeSH word for the terms you choose (see earlier discussion).
- "Citation Matcher" is useful when you are looking for a particular article and you know some of the relevant information, but not all. You may know the name of the journal, issue, author's name, or page of the journal.

Looking at the main screen, you will see an area for typing the search term. You can make a choice about how many articles you want to be displayed on the same page. You can also set date limits; for example,

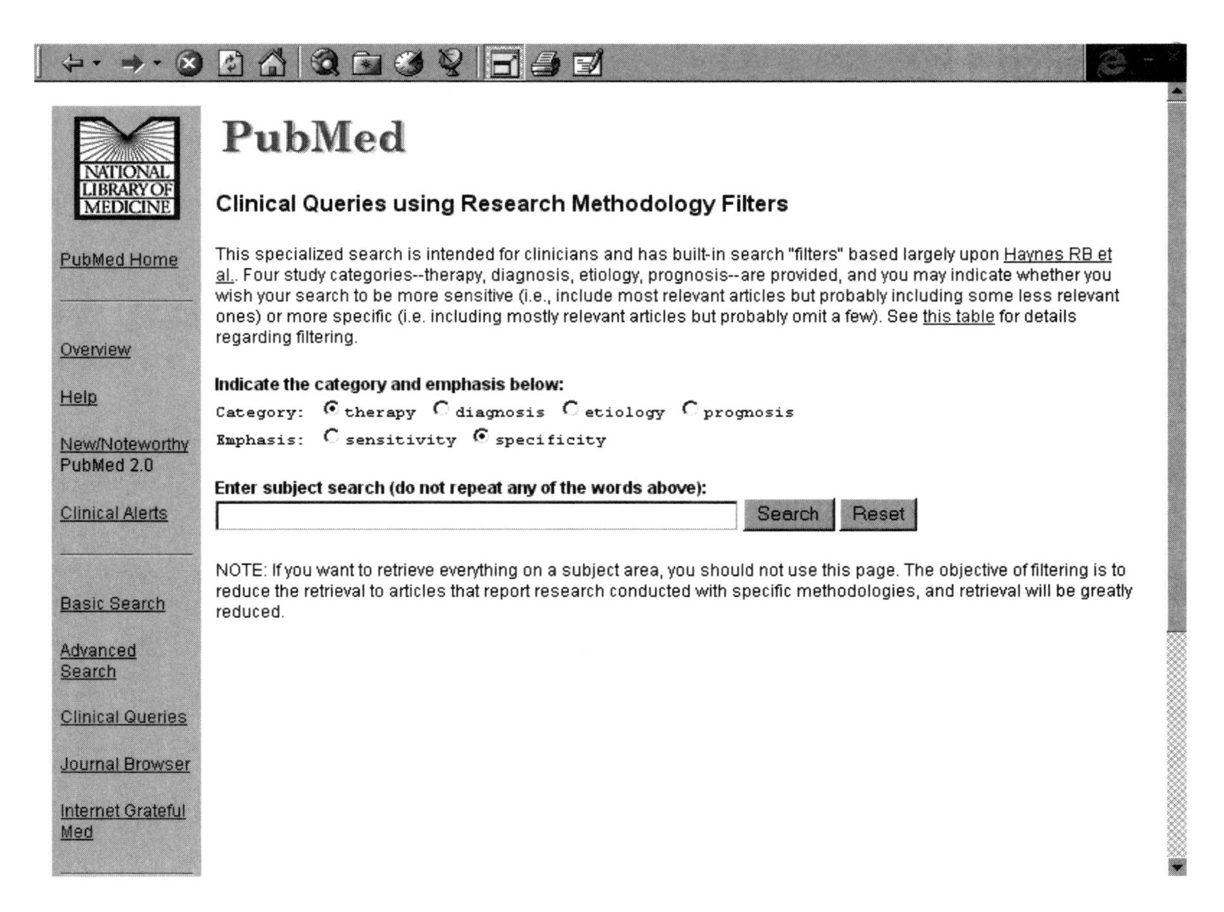

FIGURE 13–9.

whether you want to search for articles in the past 1, 5, or 10 years. You can also perform a search using Boolean logic. This is the system of logic that represents relationships between entities. There are three operators: "AND," "OR," and "NOT." "AND" is used to retrieve a set containing all terms with "AND" between them. "OR" helps retrieve a set with citations containing at least one search term out of the ones with "OR" between them. "NOT" is used to retrieve a set that excludes the term followed by "NOT." These terms should be written in capitals and should be preceded and followed by a space.

Let's look at an example. Suppose I want to search for articles on the use of beta blockers in cardiomyopathy, but I only want studies that used carvedilol or metoprolol. Furthermore, I do not want the studies that include cases with *ischemic* cardiomyopathy. The search term would be written as follows: Carvedilol OR metoprolol AND cardiomyopathy NOT ischemic. Now, I only want to see the papers published in the past year, and I want 50 papers to be displayed on the page.

This search yielded the page shown in Figure 13–10. As shown in this figure, many of the papers may have metoprolol as well as captopril. If I do not want the papers with captopril, I can narrow the search further by writing: Carvedilol OR metoprolol NOT captopril AND cardiomyopathy NOT ischemic. This screen contains the following tabs:

- "Display," which shows details of all or selected articles.
- "Order," which allows you to order papers in return for money.
- Small square boxes, to allow you to select a particular article for detailed display; you can choose more than one and see the detailed forms all at once.
- You can click on author's name to get some details individually
- "See related articles," which is self-explanatory.

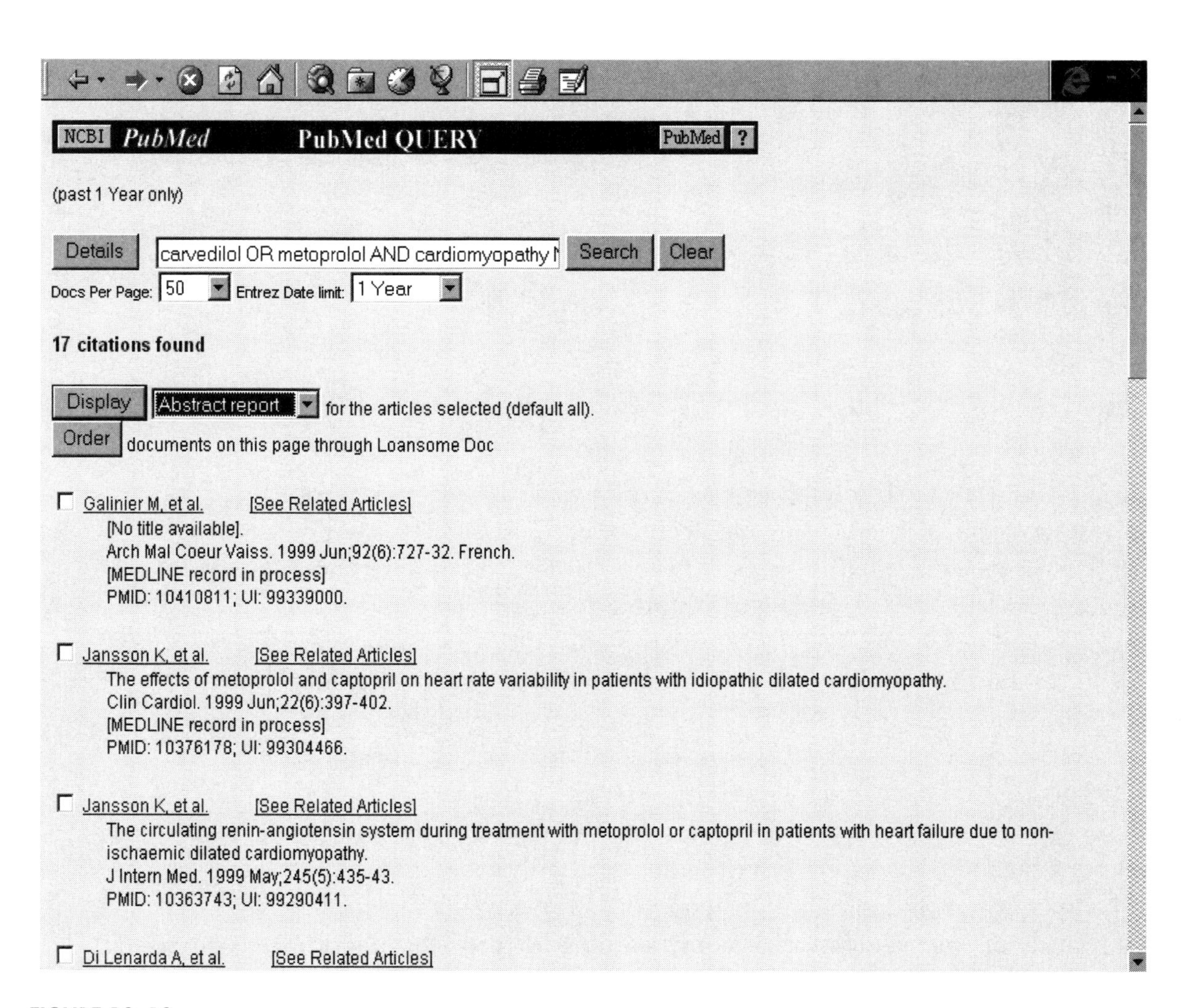

FIGURE 13–10.

Advanced Search

Clicking on the "Advanced Search" tab on the PubMed page will take you to the screen shown in Figure 13–11. This lets you specify search fields somewhat like "Apply Limits" in IGM. You can specify more than one field by repeating the same steps.

INTERNET

This system, which connects millions of computers all across the world, is a great resource for information. Once you connect your computer to the Internet, you can use different search engines or Web directories to obtain information you want. **www.yahoo.com** is one of the major Web directories.

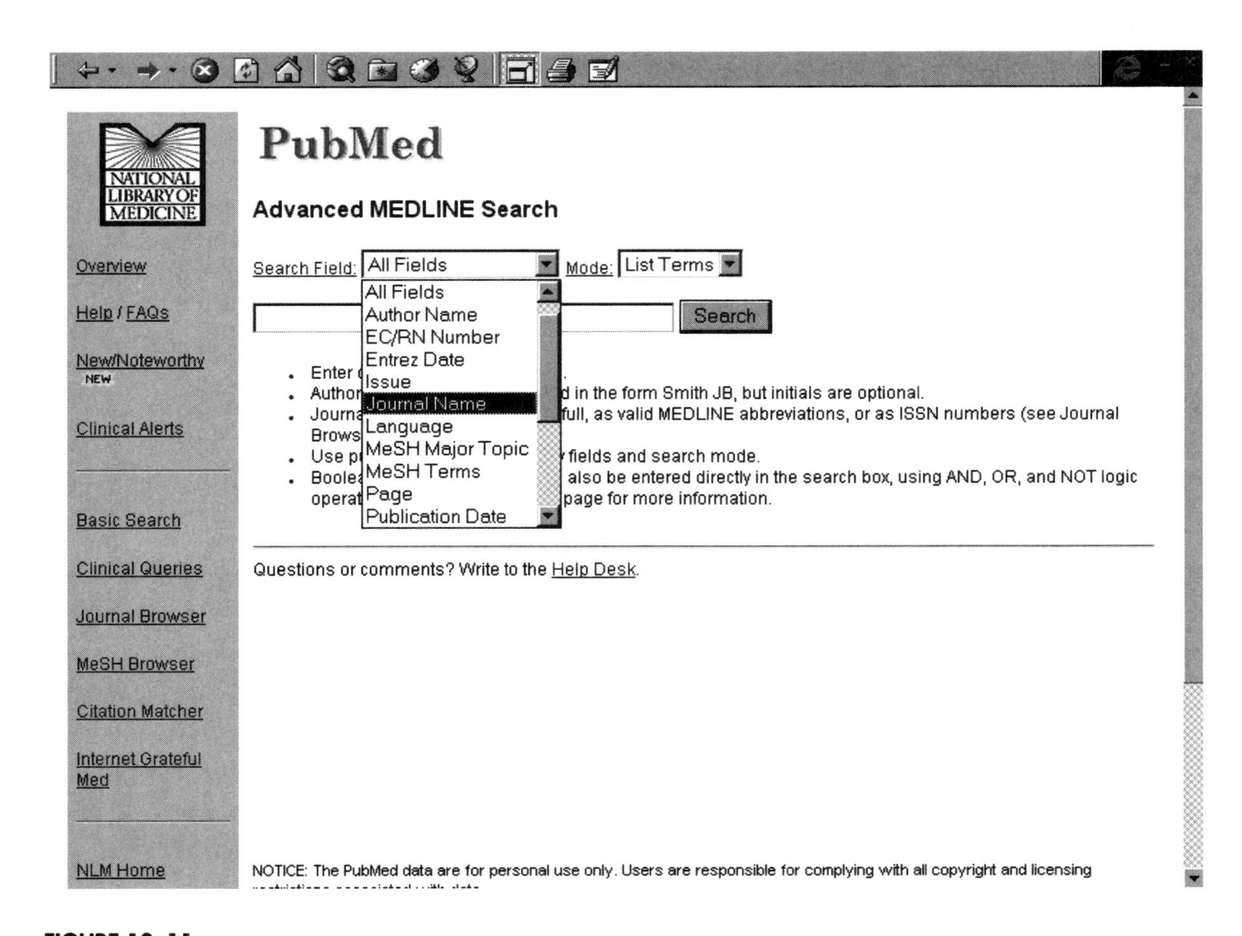

FIGURE 13–11.

Some common search engine addresses are:

www.altavista.com
www.infoseek.com
www.lycos.com
www.excite.com

You can go to the "File" tab on the computer screen, and then click on "open." This will give you an empty box where you can type one of the addresses shown above and press "Enter." From that point, you can go on to search for the topics of interest. Yahoo also offers free e-mail access. This information is meant to provide your initial introduction to Internet. Beyond that, the whole wide world of the Internet is yours to explore.

HIGHLY INFORMED PATIENTS

The Internet is a system that functions like a state of anarchy, in which anyone has the right to say whatever he or she wants. There is no guarantee about the quality of information to be found on the net. Your patients may occasionally ask you questions about something they read on the Internet. Occasionally, you will not have heard about the subject in question. As always, here too, you should be your patient's advocate and guide. Following are some important points to keep in mind:

- If you do not know what the patient is talking about, concede ignorance. Sometimes it is helpful to ask the patient to get you the source of the information to see if you can evaluate it more thoroughly.
- Show due respect to the patient's information. If you do not agree with the information, say so and present your opinion on the basis of the best available evidence.
- You may wish to guide your patients toward some reputable sources of information on the Web. One of them is the MEDLINE site called "MEDLINE plus," which will take the user to some good sources. The address is *www.nlm.nih.gov/databases/freemedl.html*.

Following are a few useful questions to help you and your patients evaluate sources of information on the net:

- ❑ Who is the author?
- ❑ Is the author the original creator of the information?
- ❑ What is the author's standing in the field of the subject that he or she is writing on?
- ❑ How frequently is the information updated?
- ❑ Could the author be biased in his or her opinion?
- ❑ Is the information evaluated before being put on the Net?

CHAPTER 14

The Second Year of Residency

FELLOWSHIP HUNTING

The majority of IMGs who come to the United States have becoming a specialist as their goal. The word "specialist" in this context means that they want to become a cardiologist, gastroentererologist, or other specialized practitioner after finishing their residency in medicine. A small number of IMGs who do a surgical residency want to go on to do further training in a subspeciality such as cardiothoracic surgery, vascular surgery, and so on. There is a lot of competition for good fellowship positions. A look at the timeline on the next pages reveals that you have to start early to be able to have a good chance of getting into a good program.

THE IMG PERSPECTIVE

Most IMGs think that research is the most important factor in getting a good fellowship.

- ❑ Most IMGs interested in a fellowship scramble to line up a research project early in the second year once they regain control of their schedule after a busy year of internship. Some of them think it to be the most important factor for getting into a fellowship.
- ❑ Some IMGs have a hard time deciding who to ask for recommendation letters.
- ❑ A significant percentage of IMGs who have succeeded in being accepted into a good fellowship do not really know what worked for them!

I went through the same drill when I was looking for a cardiology fellowship. I had 10 (if not more) people read my personal statement. I spent hours on research projects that never reached fruition. I did what I had seen my senior residents doing. One of my senior residents had gotten into a cardiology fellowship the year before I applied. I asked him what he felt had worked for him. He laughed and said, "If I ever have enough money in my life, I am going to spend a lot of it to find the answer to that question." This statement explained his confusion well, despite the jocular tone. Based on his experience, and that of many others, I think a systematic approach to fellowship hunting makes a big difference. The time-line given below should apply to the majority of fellowships.

TIMELINE

Time Frame	Actions
1. From the first day of residency	❑ Maintain good performance in your residency. ❑ Arrange to do the desired subspecialty elective in the program where you want to do your fellowship. Time this elective to precede or occur around interview time for best results.
2. July–August of second year of residency (2 years before starting the fellowship. As an example, if you are looking for a fellowship that starts in July of 2002, you should start in July–August of 2000)	❑ Request applications from different programs
3. August–September	❑ Request your recommendation letters. ❑ Write your personal statement.
4. September–October	❑ Mail applications.
5. November–December	❑ Follow up to see if your recommendation letters have been mailed. ❑ Follow up to see if your application has been received. Some program secretaries may sort out the applications late. Don't push. It can hurt your cause. Be patient and call them later.
6. December	❑ Medical Specialty Matching Program (MSMP) material becomes available. MSMP is a subdivision of NRMP that manages matching for fellowship positions. Most positions in the following specialties are filled through MSMP: cardiovascular disease, gastroenterology, infectious disease, pulmonary disease. Arrange interviews as calls are received.
7. Approximately May of second year	❑ Deadline for submitting rank order list to MSMP, if applicable.
8. June	❑ Matching results are announced. Post match scramble starts.

FACTORS INFLUENCING ACCEPTANCE INTO A FELLOWSHIP PROGRAM

I could not find much information in the published literature regarding factors that influence a candidate's chances of being accepted into the fellowship of his or her choice. However, Dr. Nasser M. Gayed did a survey in 1993 to assess the importance of different criteria used by cardiology fellowship directors in choosing fellows. An article describing the survey is available on the Web at *www.apdim.med.edu/cim/v11_2/c10.htm*. I believe we may be able to extrapolate Dr. Gayed's findings to other fellowships. According to his survey, the factors used in selecting cardiology fellows in *descending* order of relevance were:

Positive and negative comments by the residency program director are the most important factors in the selection of candidates for fellowship, according to one survey.

1. Negative comments or hints of underlying problems in the program director's letter.
2. Personal comments by the program director of internal medicine
3. The personal aspect of the interview
4. A letter of recommendation from a cardiologist known to the fellowship program director
5. The program director's letter, in general
6. The candidate's performance during his or her elective at the application site
7. Rank order in the residency class
8. Genuine interest in research
9. Being a graduate of a U.S. medical school
10. A letter of recommendation from a nationally known cardiologist
11. Doing a residency program at an institution with a well-known cardiology division
12. Participation in research prior to the fellowship
13. Assessment of medical knowledge during the interview (see also number 3)
14. Publications prior to fellowship
15. Performance on the FMGEMs (for IMGs)
16. Performance on the FLEX (if taken)
17. Performance on the American Board of Internal Medicine (ABIM) exam (if available)
18. U.S. citizenship
19. Performance on the National Board of Medical Examiners (NBME) exam

During my own research, I interviewed a number of faculty members who have been in the position of choosing fellows. The salient points that came to light follow.

- *Recommendations*. These appear to be the most important factor in most cases. Most of the persons I interviewed said, "If someone I know calls in support of a candidate, that will strongly tilt the balance in favor of that candidate." Although some of my interviewees stated that it *should* not be the major criteria, they conceded that *it is* a strong consideration.

You do not need to have scientific publications under your belt to be accepted into fellowship.

- *Research*. Most interviewees do not believe that having published in a journal is a strong factor. The candidate's interest in research is felt to be a stronger consideration. This is similar to the findings in Dr. Gayed's survey.
- *Institution of residency*. A candidate doing residency in a nationally well-known program gets a head start, say my interviewees.
- *International graduates*. I asked about special considerations in the case of an IMG applicant. It seems that the considerations are basically the same as for U.S. medical graduates. However, evaluation of the candidate's ability to communicate seems to be one of the important tasks when interviewing an IMG.

SUMMARY OF SUGGESTIONS

- If you are applying for the fellowship during residency, you should arrange to have less busy elective rotations from January to March of your second year, when most of the interviews take place. That will allow you to have time for interviews. Tell your program director and chief resident about your plans.
- The single most important factor influencing your chances of being accepted into a fellowship is the recommendations you receive from faculty in your residency program.

Choose your letter writers carefully.

- You should carefully choose the people who write your letters of recommendation. If in doubt, it is okay to ask a potential letter writter whether he or she would be able to give you a strongly supportive letter. This gives the other person a chance to wriggle out of the obligation if he or she wants to. It is an unpardonable sin to select a person who will write negative remarks about you. An intern in a typical program interacts with tens of faculty members during the year. Odds are, there are three faculty members somewhere who are ready to swear that you are the Einstein incarnate.

- Give your letter writer enough time for writing your recommendation. A well written, thoughtful letter demands a particular frame of mind and time.
- Genuine interest in research may be considered more important than either prior participation in research or previous publication. You may be able to show a burning enthusiasm for research during the interview, but before that, your personal statement and curriculum vitae should reflect that interest. This helps attract notice in a pile of applications for fellowship.
- If you have identified a program of subspecialization, request that your current program help you do an elective there. You may be able to hit the target much easier than you thought.
- No program should be considered too good to apply for. Once you receive an interview call, you start from the same point as all the other interviewees.

BECOMING A SENIOR RESIDENT

The second year of residency is not discussed much in the published literature. There is a strong awareness of the hardships faced by interns, thanks to the published material. However, the second year can also cause a lot of anxiety for some residents. On the one hand, there is a feeling of happiness that you are no longer the lowest person in the hierarchy, on the other hand there is the anxiety of becoming a "senior." Here are a few suggestions to help you deal with these new responsibilities:

Learn to be a leader and trust your team members while subtly keeping a check on quality.

- Give your interns their own breathing space. It can be difficult to suddenly start trusting others with the job that you were doing yourself. That is why you may initially be tempted to check everything yourself. Keep the intern informed of everything you are doing with his or her patients. Remember, now he or she is the patient's primary doctor.
- Sometimes you may find out something about a patient before the patient's primary doctor (your intern) does. If it demands urgent attention, take care of it yourself and let the intern know about it. Otherwise, wait until the intern sees the patient. This way you will now throw your interns off rhythm with your frequent interjections. They will appreciate you for this consideration.

- The intern is in the same position you were in a year ago. He or she is under pressure to prove capable to his or her co-workers. Let your intern do so and, if possible, help him or her on that account. Do not try to compete with your intern in the game of impressing your superiors.
- Be the leader of the team. Help find the answers to the questions that come up during patient rounds.

RESIDENT AS TEACHER

It is important to be a good teacher as a resident for the following reasons:

- Being a good teacher is a well-respected trait in the United States.
- Students and other residents look forward to learning new things during each rotation.
- A majority of interns and students feel motivated to do a reasonable amount of scut work as long as they feel they are learning.

Following are a few tips on how to be a good teacher as a resident:

- Demonstrate good physical examination techniques to your team members. All of your team members should be encouraged to invite each other to observe characteristic and atypical physical findings in patients on your team.
- Help the team by bringing up questions during rounds. The duty to find answers to these queries can be divided among all team members.
- All team members should be given topics of mutual interest on which to talk for a few minutes.
- Feel the pulse of your team. Steer your teaching attendings' discussions toward topics that are of interest to your team members.
- Do not teach just to impress or overwhelm others.

RECOMMENDED READING

Being a teacher is an important—and a fun—part of being a resident.

The following book offers several good tips on how to be a good presenter in different settings; for example, teaching rounds, morning report, bedside teaching, journal club, and so on:

Schwenk TL, Whitman N: *Residents as teachers: A guide to educational practice*, 2nd ed. (Available from Dr. Neal Whitman, Department of Family and Preventive Medicine, University of Utah School of Medicine, Salt Lake City, UT 1993.)

CHAPTER 15

The Final Year

The final year of residency is one that demands a lot of planning. Many important decisions need to be made, and one should fill in any gaps in knowledge as a part of "polishing the rough edges." Speaking from the perspective of an IMG, I have divided the chapter into the following sections:

1. Getting ready to go back home
2. Continuing with a fellowship
3. The job hunt
   a. Your visa type
   b. Your job options
   c. An IMG's job hunt
   d. Your contract—The fine print
4. Buying a house
5. Moving
6. Board certification
7. Licensing boards
8. Polishing the rough edges

GETTING READY TO GO BACK HOME

For those planning to return to their respective countries after residency training, the completion of the residency program is the culmination of their dreams. Some suggestions pertinent to these individuals were given in Chapter 1. Some additional tips follow.

1. The U.S. degree is highly respected throughout the world. You should be aware of the value of your achievement. That will help you sell yourself better.

2. Your attitude is totally different as compared to when you came here. You will have different (read that as better) expectations of yourself.
3. Your return to your country should be very well planned. It is worthwhile to visit your country before your final return after finishing your studies. You have a greater bargaining power while you are still in the United States because the people with whom you interview will not know whether you might opt to stay in the United States.
4. You should not limit your search to only a few places. Look around for the best deal before you drop your anchor.
5. Research the possibility of taking medical instruments back with you. Inquire about the laws in the United States and your own country governing import and export. Your visa status may have a bearing on the application of these laws.

Secure a job in your chosen place before leaving the United States for good.

CONTINUING WITH A FELLOWSHIP

If you are going to do a fellowship, your financial situation is not likely to change much. For all practical purposes, this will be an extension of your residency. For those leaving to go to another area, moving is the major issue. Before deciding to move for a fellowship, you should have already made arrangements for your spouse's employment prospects and your child's schooling.

THE JOB HUNT

IMGs constituted 23.3 percent of the total number of physicians in the United States in 1997. Several considerations that apply specifically to IMGs are worth mentioning here. Let me start with a point that is lopsidedly in favor of IMGs. Most United States medical graduates leave medical school with loans of $100 to $150 thousand hanging over their heads. The major part of this loan accrues as a result of the tuition fee for medical school. These U.S. graduates have to start paying off their loans. Most IMGs have no such financial obligations.

Another point worth mentioning concerns networking. A very high percentage of American graduates report that they get their job through personal contacts. This is even more important for IMGs. You have a good opportunity during your residency to work with and evaluate the work styles of many different people. Similarly, you are watched by a lot of people. This is a good place to forge mutually useful partnerships and contacts.

YOUR VISA TYPE

- ❑ If you are a green card holder or a U.S. citizen, you do not have to do any more paperwork in this field.
- ❑ If you have an H-1 visa, you have to find an employer that is ready to sponsor you for this visa. At the time of the writing of this book, H-1 visa holders can stay in the United States for a maximum of 6 years. You have to obtain a green card before the end of that time if you wish to stay on in the country. Once an H-1 visa holding physician lands a job, he or she has to go through labor certification before applying for a green card. This can be a lengthy process. One way to cut the bureaucratic red tape is the "national interest waiver" petition. Talk to a good immigration lawyer about the different options available to you.
- ❑ If you came here on a J-1 visa, you are obliged to return to the country of your last permanent residence for 2 years before you can apply for a job in the United States (if you want to). There are some options available if you want to try to obtain a waiver of this condition. Again, this is an ever-changing field, and you should check with a good immigration lawyer.

YOUR JOB OPTIONS

I touched on this subject in Chapter 1 under the heading of "Goal Setting." Here are some additional points regarding the different types of practice options available to you.

Hospitalist

In this type of practice, you only take care of patients in an inpatient setting. You are not the primary doctor to the patient in the real sense of that term. The patient sees another doctor as an outpatient before or after this hospital admission. "Hospitalist" is a new term first coined in the *New England Journal of Medicine* in 1996. You may want to learn more about this style of practice before you make up your mind about your future course. The National Association of Inpatient Physicians has a Web site at *www.naiponline.org*.

Working with Health Maintenance Organizations (HMOs)

Managed care organizations are taking over a bigger and bigger chunk of the health care market in the United States. As a result, a lot of physicians now work in association with some HMOs. There are several different ways in which you could practice in association with an HMO.

Staff Model HMO. The physicians in this model are hired directly by the HMO to take care of its patients.

Group Model HMO. This may be further classified as "captive" or "independent." In the captive model, the HMO forms a group, mostly a multispecialty one, to provide care to its patients. In the independent model, the HMO contracts with an existing group for the care of its patients.

Network Model HMO. In this model, the HMO contracts with different physicians in the community to provide care to its patients for a predefined amount per member. The physician may continue with his or her own practice apart from seeing the patients that come with the HMO contract. This has the potential to be a losing proposition as you are providing total care to the patient for a predefined sum.

Independent Practice Association (IPA). In this model, physicians form an intermediary organization that contracts with payers to provide services for a negotiated rate.

You should evaluate the pros and cons of these styles of practice. You should also assess the financial condition of a managed care organization before signing on with it. There have been many instances of physicians sinking along with financially unsound organizations.

AN IMG'S JOB HUNT

An IMG's options in job hunting can change according to the type of visa he or she holds. The paperwork involved in sponsoring a physician holding a J-1 or H-1 visa can be enormous and intimidating to the inexperienced employer. You should be prepared to start your job search more than a year in advance. Sometimes if you educate your potential employer about the paperwork, he or she may become interested in going the extra mile for you.

You have a better chance of getting a good job through personal contacts than through other avenues. Carefully evaluate the credentials of persons who claim to "specialize" in getting jobs for physicians with J-1 or H-1 visas. Many IMGs have related stories of exploitation at the workplace and unkept promises after being charged a lot of money. Other classic methods available for job hunting include:

1. Classified ads in the major medical journals
2. Recruiters: You should carefully evaluate a recruiter before assigning to this person the important responsibility of finding a job for you. It is better to choose someone who has worked satisfactorily for another person who is well known to you. Beware of ads that give a P.O. box and no contact number. Some big institutions have recruiters on their payroll. These persons do headhunting for these institutions. Some database companies will provide the service of circulating your CV to potential employers.

Current Procedural Terminology (CPT) Tangles

All the services provided by physicians are classified by codes called CPT codes. Physicians or hospitals are paid according to these codes. It is very important that you learn these codes for the following reasons:

It is important to learn about CPT codes before getting into practice, and residency is the best time to learn.

- A wrong code charged for a service can constitute a fraud that can ruin one's professional career.
- A good knowledge of this system helps you do proper documentation on the billing sheets. This can be helpful evidence whenever you happen to be audited by a paying agency such as Medicare, Medicaid, or the patient's insurance agency.

Every medical resident in the United States sees patients at an ambulatory clinic. This is a good place to learn how to fill out billing sheets for the patients that you see. The final year is the time to pay special attention to this issue. Apart from other characteristics, the knowledge of this aspect of practice will definitely endear you to your employer and his or her billing department.

Other ways of learning this task are through in-house training sessions or by working with billing department staff. Many institutions offer free seminars on CPT codes to their employees. Residents are usually welcome to these sessions. Each hospital has a billing department with employees who specialize in this area. These people never come into direct contact with residents. They are behind-the-scene operators. However, these people can be your great resource while learning your way around the CPT tangles.

YOUR CONTRACT—THE FINE PRINT

I am talking about the contract you will sign with your employer after finishing your residency. A survey of IMGs going into practice has brought the following concerns to light:

Always have a professional read over your contract.

- Most IMGs do not have their contract read over by a professional specializing in contract law. They may feel embarrassed about being "cheap" with a "friend" (the employer). The problem is that in case of a dispute, the contract with its language full of legalese is the item upon which the discussion will hinge.
- Some IMGs, especially those without a green card or citizenship, do not feel that they are in a position to negotiate. There is nothing farther from truth than this. No contract is ever written to be carved in granite. There is always a room for negotiation, but the time for that is *before* you sign the contract. One of my mentors, my fellowship program director, Dr. Collins, always says, "You will never know what you could get unless you ask for it."

Suggestions for Reviewing Your Contract

- Never have a "we will see" attitude towards different clauses of the contract that exist only in your dreams. For all practical purposes, if a thing is not written in the contract, it does not happen.
- Seeking a professional's opinion and acting on it does not constitute being "cheap" to a "friend." Your employer did not write the contract. A professional did this for him or her.
- You carefully review the type of malpractice insurance offered by an employer. Sometimes a doctor is sued at a time much later than the time of service. In the "claims made" type of insurance, your

insurance will cover your malpractice claims only if the company that insured you at the time of the alleged occurrence is the same as the one at the time of suit. In contrast, "occurrence made" insurance will cover all the claims that arise out of the services provided during the time that the insurance carrier was the provider. If you have "claims made" insurance, you should buy an insurance "tail." This covers claims in the event that you have changed carriers between the occurrence and the time of suit. You will have to negotiate who will buy the insurance tail. You should also read the fine print of your insurance coverage. The data on median professional liability premiums and coverage limits for various specialties are available in the following book: Gonzalez ML, Zhang P (eds): *Physician Marketplace Statistics 1997/1998*. Chicago: American Medical Association, 1998.

- ❑ Pay particular attention to the life and disability insurance package offered by prospective employers.

BUYING A HOUSE

Evaluate your financial situation critically before jumping in to buy the biggest house available.

Getting a well-paying job after years of hard work is the realization of one of your dreams. Buying a nice, big house is another dream of most physicians. It is very easy to get carried away by the push to try to buy a big house that reflects your new status. You should always evaluate your situation and see what you can easily afford. Tips include:

- ❑ Try to put as much money as possible into your down payment. The down payment is the money that you pay at the time you purchase the house. The remainder (the cost of the house minus the down payment) is usually acquired through a loan (the mortgage). You have to pay this loan in installments along with interest charges. It makes good sense to put down as much of your own money as possible because it will decrease the amount of the loan on which you are paying interest. Some lenders may let you have a loan for the purchase of a house with as little as a 5 percent down payment. You should also have an additional 3 to 6 percent set aside to pay the closing costs, which cover the paperwork involved in buying property.
- ❑ Your monthly mortgage payment for the house should not exceed 28% of your gross monthly income.

MOVING

Moving can be accomplished in any of the following ways.

- You can rent trucks from one of the nationwide truck rental companies that you then drive to your destination. Once you reach your destination, you then return the truck to their subsidiary at the point of arrival.
- You can send boxed belongings via a carrier such as UPS that offers delivery throughout the United States at a reasonable price.
- You can hire professional movers. Be warned that moving and storage companies are one of the businesses most often reported to the Better Business Bureau (BBB). It is common to be quoted one price by a mover initially and then asked to pay more money around the time of moving. At that point, you may not have much choice but to give in. It is always a good idea to check with your local BBB about any complaints against the movers with whom you are thinking of contracting. There is a useful Web site run by the national BBB at *www.bbb.org*.

Exercise great caution when dealing with movers.

BOARD CERTIFICATION

In the present practice scenario, being board certified looks to be more of a necessity than an option.

After completing your residency in a particular field, the next step is to become board certified in that specialty. This is not an essential step prior to practice, but more and more employers now prefer board-certified physicians. Some important facts

- Some IMGs may have a visa that is limited to the time of residency training. However, there is a provision for extending the visa so that you can take the specialty board exam before leaving the United States.
- The board exam is easier to prepare for if you work toward it over a period of time rather than trying to cram for it at the eleventh hour.
- Some programs have some teaching sessions set aside for the board review topics. You should make sure that your program has such arrangement.
- Form study groups with your peers to discuss board review topics. You may have more free time in your third year with fewer on-call responsibilities. Utilize this time for discussions of topics relevant to the boards.

- There are plenty of board review courses. Nearly all good training programs should pay for such a course. You should not expect that these courses will help you learn everything in *Harrison's* in 5 or 6 days; however, they may help you fill in missing pieces of information in your knowledge base and can help you assess your level of preparation.

LICENSING BOARDS

You have to obtain a license to practice in the state in which you are planning to work. Licensure can be a lengthy process, so you should try to start early.

POLISHING THE ROUGH EDGES

The final year is the time when you have to get ready to swim with the sharks in the real world of practice. This is when you must assess yourself critically and polish any rough edges. You should determine if there are any medical or nonmedical topics that you are not comfortable with. Talk to your mentors and teachers. This may be the last time you are treated as a student. Come July 1, you may become another competitor in the wild world of practice.

Appendix

IMPORTANT ORGANIZATIONS AND AGENCIES

ACCREDITATION COUNCIL FOR GRADUATES MEDICAL EDUCATION (ACGME)

As the name implies, this is an accrediting agency. One of its parts is the Residency Review Committee (RRC) that reviews the standards of residency training programs in the United States.

> ***Telephone:*** 312-464-4920
> ***Fax:*** 312-464-4098
> ***Web site:*** *www.acgme.org*

AGENCY FOR HEALTH CARE POLICY AND RESEARCH (AHCPR)

This agency is a part of the U.S. Department of Health and Human Services. It is the lead agency supporting research designed to test the quality of health care, reduce its cost, and broaden access to essential services. AHCPR offers several useful publications, including some management guidelines, which are available free of cost.

> ***Telephone:*** Clearinghouse for publications: 800-358-9295
> ***Web site:*** *www.ahcpr.gov*

AMERICAN BOARD OF INTERNAL MEDICINE (ABIM)

This board administers certifying exams for internists and subspecialists. It also disseminates useful publications as enumerated in Chapter 12. IMGs who are eligible to finish their medicine or subspecialty training in a shorter period on the basis of previous experience have to get permission from ABIM.

Address: ABIM
501 Walnut Street, Suite 1700
Philadelphia, PA 19106-3699
Telephone: 215-446-3500; ***toll-free*** (from within the United States): 800-441-2246
Fax: 215-446-3470
Web site: *www.abim.org*

ASSOCIATION OF AMERICAN MEDICAL COLLEGES (AAMC)

This is an agency composed of various U.S. and Canadian medical schools, major teaching hospitals, health systems, veterans administration medical centers, academic and professional societies, medical students, and residents.

Web site: *www.aamc.org*

EDUCATIONAL COMMISSION FOR MEDICAL GRADUATES (ECFMG)

This is a nonprofit organization that assesses the readiness of IMGs to enter residency or fellowship in a U.S. program accredited by ACGME. It does so by certifying IMGs. At the time of the writing of this book, the steps to obtain certification are USMLE steps 1 and 2, TOEFL, and CSA. ECFMG also sponsors IMGs for a J-1 visa.

Address: ECFMG
3624, Market Street, 4th floor
Philadelphia, PA 19104-2685
Telephone: 215-386-5900
Web site: *www.ecfmg.org*

ELECTRONIC RESIDENCY APPLICATION SERVICE (ERAS)

This is the agency that electronically transmits your residency application for the specialties that go through ERAS. This has replaced, for most residencies, the paper applications that used to be sent in the past.

Web site: *www.aamc.org/eras/start.htm.*

FEDERATION OF STATE MEDICAL BOARDS (FSMB)

This is a 69-member board whose primary responsibility and obligation is to protect the public through the regulation of physicians and other health care providers. It controls licensure for the practice of medicine in the United States.

Address: FSMB, Inc.
Federal Place
400 Fuller Wiser Road, Suite 300
Euless, TX 76039
Telephone: 817-868-4000
Fax: 817-868-4099
Web site: *www.fsmb.org.*
E-mail address for inquiries regarding USMLE 3:
USMLE@fsmb.org

FELLOWSHIP AND RESIDENCY ELECTRONIC INTERACTIVE DATABASE (FREIDA)

This is a great database on the Web that provides information on graduate medical education programs, specialty status, and the physician workforce.

Web site: *www.ama-assn.org/cgi-bin/freida/freida.cgi*

HEALTH CARE FINANCING ADMINISTRATION (HCFA)

This is the government agency that administers the Medicare and Medicaid programs, which provide health care to about 25 percent of Americans. It decides the financial disbursements to doctors or the hospitals for the services provided.
Web site: *www.hcfa.gov*

NATIONAL BOARD OF MEDICAL EXAMINERS (NBME)

This board prepares and administers qualifying exams either independently or jointly with other organizations.

Telephone: 215-590-9500
Fax: 215-590-9555
Web site: *www.nbme.org*

NATIONAL RESIDENCY MATCHING PROGRAM (NRMP)

This is a private, not-for-profit entity that provides an impartial venue for matching applicants' and programs' preferences for residency.

Address: NRMP
2501 M Street N.W., Suite 1
Washington, DC 20037-1307
Telephone: 202-828-0566
Web site: *www.aamc.org/nrmp*

UNITED STATES INFORMATION AGENCY (USIA)

This is a government agency whose functions include international educational and cultural exchanges.

Address: USIA, Office of Public Liaison
301, 4th Street S.W., Room 602
Washington DC 20547
Telephone: 202-619-4355
Web site: *www.usia.gov*

UNITED STATES MEDICAL LICENSING EXAMINATION (USMLE)

This is a certifying exam governed by members from ECFMG, FSMB (Federation of State Medical Boards), NBME (National Board of Medical Examiners), and members of the public.

Address: USMLE
Office of Secretariat
3750 Market Street
Philadelphia, PA 19104
Telephone: 215-590-9600
Fax: 215-590-9470
Web site: *www.usmle.org*

UNITED STATES STATE DEPARTMENT; THE SECRETARY OF STATE

The official Web site gives useful information regarding different visas.

Web site: *www.state.gov*

WEB ADDRESSES

- **TOEFL:** *www.toefl.org*
- **American Medical Association:** *www.ama-assn.org*
- **American College of Physicians:** *www.acponline.org*
- **Sites to obtain free e-mail accounts** (please read their terms and conditions carefully): *www.yahoo.com*, *www.hotmail.com*

Index

ISBN 0-07-134724-0
90000
9 780071 347242